THE NEW BIBLE
NEW
CURE
FOR STRESS

THE NEW BIBLE CURE FOR STRESS

DON COLBERT, MD

SILOAM

Most Charisma House Book Group products are available at special quantity discounts for bulk purchase for sales promotions, premiums, fund-raising, and educational needs. For details, write Charisma House Book Group, 600 Rinehart Road, Lake Mary, Florida 32746, or telephone (407) 333-0600.

The New Bible Cure for Stress by Don Colbert, MD
Published by Siloam
Charisma Media/Charisma House Book Group
600 Rinehart Road
Lake Mary, Florida 32746
www.charismahouse.com

Unless otherwise noted, all Scripture quotations are from the Holy Bible, New Living Translation, copyright © 1996, 2004. Used by permission of Tyndale House Publishers, Inc., Wheaton, IL 60189. All rights reserved.

Scripture quotations marked kjv are from the King James Version of the Bible.

Scripture quotations marked nkjv are from the New King James Version of the Bible. Copyright © 1979, 1980, 1982 by Thomas Nelson, Inc., publishers. Used by permission.

Cover design by Nathan Morgan
Design Director: Bill Johnson

Visit the author's website at www.drcolbert.com.

Library of Congress Cataloging-in-Publication Data:
Colbert, Don.
  The new Bible cure for stress / Don Colbert.
      p. cm.
  Includes bibliographical references.
  ISBN 978-1-59979-868-4 (trade paper) -- ISBN 978-1-61638-429-6
(e-book) 1. Stress (Psychology)--Religious aspects--Christianity.

2. Stress management--Religious aspects--Christianity. 3. Stress (Psychology) 4. Stress management. I. Title.

BV4509.5.C63 2011

155.9'042--dc22

2011004675

CONTENTS

vii

A BRAND-NEW BIBLE CURE
FOR A BRAND-NEW YOU!

FEELING STRESSED OUT? It's no wonder! You and I may be living in one of the most stressful times in recent history. Daily you are being forced to cope with an onslaught of political fear and insecurity, financial uncertainty, job layoffs, constantly increasing job demands, increasing debt, relationship pressures, and much, much more. If stress is making you feel like a kettle that has reached its boiling point, then you've come to the right place. There is hope for you! You really can conquer stress and its overwhelming mental and physical effects.

By picking up this Bible Cure book, you have taken an exciting first step toward successfully surviving and conquering stress and reclaiming control over your spiritual, emotional, and physical health. Right now you may be confronting some of the greatest challenges of your life. But by understanding some of the real root causes of your stressed-out feelings, you can rise to a new level of physical, emotional, and spiritual health and joy in God.

God revealed His divine will for each of us through the apostle Paul, who wrote, "Casting all your care upon Him, for He cares for you" (1 Pet. 5:7, NKJV). Surely when we are stressed out, we are

1

missing God's best for us. But how? A closer look will reveal some hopeful answers.

ADDRESSING THE SPIRITUAL ROOTS OF DISEASE

As a Christian medical doctor I've studied and prayed about the causes of disease, and increasingly I've discovered that many diseases have very strong spiritual, mental, and emotional roots. If you are familiar with my books, then doubtless you are aware that I believe in the health of the entire person: body, mind, and spirit. Although traditional medicine often sees these facets of our being as very separate, in truth they are not. A vital link exists between the spirit, soul, and body. And although much of the disease and physical pain we suffer comes from the body, often these distresses begin in the soul, which encompasses the mind, will, and emotions.

Therefore, truly living in the divine health that God intends for us requires that we look a little deeper, beyond the physical process of disease, to the spiritual, emotional, and mental roots. I trust that you will find these pages extremely enlightening as you gain new insight and revelation to help you live your life in the robust, joyful, peaceful state of good health that God desires for you.

STRESS AND YOUR HEALTH

Surveys and research over the past two decades reveal these startling statistics concerning stress:

- Forty-three percent of all adults suffer adverse health effects due to stress.[1]

- Seventy-five to 90 percent of all visits to primary care physicians are for stress-related complaints or disorders.[2]

- Americans are consuming approximately five billion tranquilizers, five billion barbiturates, three billion amphetamines, and sixteen tons of aspirin every year.[3] Much of this medicine is taken to relieve stress or the pain associated with stress.

- Chronic stress has been linked to many leading causes of death in the United States, including cardiovascular disease, cancer, lung ailments, accidents, and suicide.

- On an average workday an estimated one million workers are absent because of stress-related complaints. Stress is said to be responsible for more than half of the 550 million workdays lost annually because of absenteeism.[4]

- A three-year study conducted by a large corporation showed that 60 percent of employee absences were due to psychological problems such as stress.[5]

Today, the negative results of stress are at an all-time high. But you do not have to sit back and become one more stress statistic. With God's help, you can fight back and win. So, as you begin to read through the pages of this book, get ready to feel better!

Originally published as *The Bible Cure for Stress* in 2002, *The New Bible Cure for Stress* has been revised and updated with the latest medical research on stress. If you compare it side by side with the previous edition, you will see that it's also larger, allowing me to expand greatly upon the information provided in the previous edition and to provide you with a deeper understanding of what you face and how to overcome it.

Unchanged from the previous edition are the timeless, life-changing, and healing scriptures throughout this book that will strengthen and encourage your spirit and soul. The proven principles, truths, and guidelines in these passages anchor the practical and medical insights also contained in this book. They will effectively focus your prayers, thoughts, and actions so you can step into God's plan of divine health for you—a plan that includes victory over stress.

Another change since the original *The Bible Cure for Stress* was published is that I've released a book called *The Seven Pillars of Health.* I encourage you to read it because the principles of health it contains are the foundation to healthy living that will affect all areas of your life. It sets the stage for everything you will ever read in any other book I've published—including this one. Because the topic of stress affects so many people, I've also released a book called *Stress Less*, which expands even further on my principles of stress management and offers you a way to live in health and peace.

There is much you can do to rise above stress and its negative health impact upon your life. You really can stand up and face the challenges of stress with fresh confidence, renewed determination, and the wonderful knowledge that God is real, that He is alive, and that His power is greater than any other force in the universe.

It is my prayer that these powerful strategies for conquering stress will bring health, wholeness, and spiritual refreshing to you—body, mind, and spirit. May they deepen your fellowship with God and strengthen your ability to worship and serve Him.

—DON COLBERT, MD

A BIBLE CURE Prayer for You

Dear heavenly Father, You created me, and You are well aware of the pressures and emotional turmoil that surround me every day. As I read through this Bible Cure book, give me a special grace to rise up to a bold new level of faith and courage in You.

God, I thank You that before my circumstances were ever set in motion, You had created a plan for my victory over them. Thank You for Your wonderful Word, which promises special protection and deliverance when I am tempted to feel overwhelmed by stressful circumstances. Thank You for making it possible for me to walk in Your divine health for my total being—body, mind, and spirit—free from the physical and emotional ravages of stress. In Jesus's name, amen.

Chapter 1

UNDERSTANDING THE ROOTS OF STRESS

THE BIBLE SAYS, "People judge by outward appearance, but the LORD looks at the heart" (1 Sam. 16:7). In other words, God looks far beyond what people see, for He is able to see the very root of a problem.

Often I meet people who complain about the modern medical profession. They tell me that their doctors seem to usually treat symptoms with a variety of drugs, but seldom do they attempt to discover the root causes. Under the present medical system in America, today's physicians often can be left feeling like little more than legal drug dispensers.

God promises us that if we seek, we will find; if we knock, the door will open to us (Luke 11:9). He promises to give us wisdom and understanding; all we must do is ask Him for it. To understand and overcome stress, I believe it is extremely important to go beyond simple pharmaceutical remedies, such as Prozac and Xanax, that merely mask the symptoms.

What would happen if the red oil light in your car was on and you took it to a mechanic to have the warning light turned off? The annoying problem has been alleviated, but the root could remain. In time, the problem would grow much worse, creating even more serious problems. Before long, your engine could be destroyed because you only treated the symptoms and never discovered the root cause.

Your body is similar. Stress is little more than a symptom of something much more serious lying right beneath the surface of your life. If you don't discover the root of your stress, eventually you could develop chronic diseases.

So, let's dig a little deeper to begin to understand how stressed out you really are.

> So I say, let the Holy Spirit guide your lives. Then you won't be doing what your sinful nature craves.
> —GALATIANS 5:16

WHAT IS STRESS?

The dictionary defines *stress* as "mental or physical tension or strain." In my opinion, stress is simply the pressures of life and how one perceives, reacts, and copes with those pressures.

We have mentioned that chronic stress has been linked to many diseases, including cardiovascular disease, high blood pressure, spastic colon, tension headaches, ulcers, cancer, chronic fatigue, insomnia, depression, anxiety, strokes, asthma, skin rashes, arrhythmias, panic attacks, autoimmune diseases, and much more.

Stressful feelings are very often the result of:

- Demands placed upon us by everyday life
- Major lifestyle changes with which we must deal

According to the American Psychological Association Survey in 2007, Americans are more stressed over work and money than anything else. The following graph shows the results of the APA poll of 1,848 people. Participants were read a list of stressors, and the following percentages indicate how many times each stressor was identified as a "very significant source" of stress.[1]

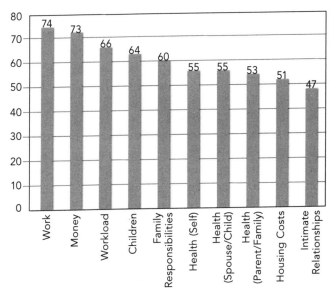

While work is the number one stressor, another one of the most stressful life events you can face is the loss of employment and mounting debt. In recent years, unemployment has skyrocketed. It's much harder to find a job right now than it was when I published the first edition of this book in 2002. If recently you've lost a job or know someone who has, then you are well aware of the stress involved. In times of financial uncertainty, learning a strategy to help you cope with stress can be a lifesaver. I recommend books by Dave Ramsey and Crown Financial Ministries, which are taught at many churches. I also recommend that you begin confessing the affirmations for favor and financial blessing in Appendix A of this book. Read on for more powerful information that can get you through this challenging period of time.

A BIBLE CURE Health Tip
A Life-Event Test

Take this life-event test to determine how the changes in your lifestyle affect your stress levels as compared to others. You may be surprised to discover how much your lifestyle changes have affected the levels of stress in your life.[2]

__ Death of a spouse (or child)	100
__ Divorce	73
__ Marital separation	65
__ Jail term	63
__ Death of close family member	63
__ Personal injury or illness	53
__ Marriage	50
__ Fired at work	47
__ Marital reconciliation	45
__ Retirement	45
__ Change in family member's health	44
__ Pregnancy	40
__ Sex difficulties	39

__ Addition to family	39
__ Business readjustment	39
__ Change in financial state	38
__ Death of close friend	37
__ Change to different line of work	36
__ Change in number of marital arguments	35
__ Mortgage or loan for major purchases	31
__ Foreclosure of mortgage or loan	30
__ Change in work responsibilities	29
__ Son or daughter leaving home	29
__ Trouble with in-laws	29
__ Outstanding personal achievement	28
__ Spouse begins or stops work	26
__ Starting or finishing school	26
__ Change in living conditions	25
__ Revision of personal habits	24
__ Trouble with boss	23
__ Change in work hours, conditions	20
__ Change in residence	20
__ Change in schools	20
__ Change in recreational habits	19
__ Change in church activities	19
__ Change in social activities	18
__ Loan for minor purchase (car, TV, etc.)	17
__ Change in sleeping habits	16
__ Change in number of family gatherings	15
__ Change in eating habits	15

__ Vacation	13
__ Christmas season	12
__ Minor violations of the law	11

Total score_____

Now, add up the point values of all the items you checked. If your score is 300 or more, according to statistics you stand an almost 80 percent chance of getting sick in the near future. If your score is 150 to 299, your chances of becoming ill are about 50 percent. If your score is less than 150, your chance of illness is about 30 percent.

HOW DID YOU SCORE?

Well, how did you score? Do you have more stress-producing life events than you might have guessed? Even if your score was lower than you anticipated, your score does not necessarily indicate how YOU, as an individual, feel and react to stress. Stress is a very individualistic experience.

HOW YOU REACT

Not everyone reacts to the same circumstances by feeling the same degree of stress. One person might go skydiving for fun and relaxation, while for another this experience would feel like the most stressful time of his or her life. Since one person's stress can be another person's pleasure, we see that stress is a result of how we as individuals interpret the events in our world. Perception is everything when it comes to stress. We cannot always control the many stressful circumstances that surround our lives, but we can control our perception of them, and we can control our reactions to those events. Understanding how to deal with the root causes of stress is a vital key to managing stress. I investigate this further in my books *Stress Less, Deadly Emotions,* and *The New Bible Cure for Depression and Anxiety.*

A **BIBLE CURE** Health Tip
Avoid Distortional Thinking

Many times a stressful situation is compounded when people listen to their own negative or distorted thought patterns as they try to deal with the situation. I sometimes call this "stinking thinking." The next time you find yourself in a stressful situation, try to avoid the following negative thought processes that can lead to distortional thinking.

- *Worst case scenarios.* Don't let your imagination run wild and create mountains out of molehills. Focus on what you *know* and ask God for wisdom in how you should handle it.

- *"Awfulizing."* This is my term for what happens when people immediately give a situation an "awful" or "terrible" label. Instead, notice the difference when you say it is "unfortunate" or "inconvenient" and put the proper perspective on the situation.

- *"Should" statements.* These are unenforceable rules that we place on others but have no authority to enforce. Therefore, they create stress. For example, if someone cuts in line in front of you, it is likely to create stress if you think, "You should not cut in line." Instead, give the gift of mercy, and stress melts away. Resist the urge to start placing blame with "should" statements.

- *"What if" thinking.* This kind of thinking can stress people
  for years on end. The problem with "what if" thinking
  is that you usually start expecting and anticipating all
  negative outcomes, which creates even more stress as you
  try to figure out what to do if a bad outcome occurs. Stop
  worrying about "what if" and ask God for divine wisdom
  and revelation regarding your problem. Philippians 4:6–7
  says it best: "Be anxious for nothing, but in everything
  by prayer and supplication, with thanksgiving, let your
  requests be made known to God; and the peace of God,
  which surpasses all understanding, will guard your hearts
  and minds through Christ Jesus" (NKJV).

Good vs. Bad Stress—Too Much vs. Too Little

It may surprise you to learn that not all stress is bad. In fact,
some stress is very beneficial. What determines whether it's good
or bad is *how much* stress you are under. A little stress can be
good, but too much stress can be very bad.

Stress is similar to the tuning of guitar strings. Just the right
amount of pressure on the tuning peg of the guitar is required
to gain the desired sound. Too little stress on those guitar
strings creates a negative effect. Without some tension on the
strings, the music sounds horrible. Similarly, too little stress in
your life can leave you feeling bored, restless, understimulated
and unable to perform adequately.

But if you pull those guitar strings too tightly, they can
break. In the same way, too much stress in your life can cause
you to perform poorly, creating anxiety, nervousness, depression,

irritability, forgetfulness, problems concentrating, problems making decisions, and many health problems.

This happens when the pressures of life exceed your ability to cope. This "bad" or excessive stress can be either too much stress of the acute or short-term variety, or it can be stress for too long a time—the chronic or long-term variety.

A **BIBLE CURE** *Health Tip*
Physical Results of Excessive Stress

As I explain in my book *Stress Less*, excessive stress is extremely damaging to the human body and predisposes a person to develop:

- Cardiovascular disease and hypertension, elevated cholesterol levels, arrhythmias (abnormal heart rhythms), mitral valve prolapse, and palpitations, as well as heart attack and stroke
- Skin eruptions such as seborrhea, eczema, hives, psoriasis, and even acne
- GI disorders such as irritable bowel syndrome, gastroesophageal reflux disease, gastritis, ulcers, and inflammatory bowel disease (such as ulcerative colitis and Crohn's disease)
- Autoimmune diseases such as rheumatoid arthritis, lupus, and multiple sclerosis
- Genitourinary problems including impotence, infertility, chronic prostatitis, recurrent urinary tract infections, recurrent yeast infections, imbalance of sex hormones, decreased sex drive, and frequent urination

- Immune impairments that lead to chronic and recurrent ear infections, colds, sinus infections, sore throats, bouts with the flu, bronchitis, or pneumonia, as well as chronic and recurring infections of all types

- Pain and inflammatory conditions such as tendonitis, migraine and tension headaches, carpal tunnel syndrome, TMJ problems, fibromyalgia, chronic back pain, and other chronic pain syndromes

- Other ailments, including chemical sensitivities, chronic allergies (both environmental and food), and chronic fatigue

Chronic stress has been shown to slowly erode bone mass and may eventually lead to osteoporosis.

Long-term stress can affect a person's mental state and has been known to cause memory loss. Chronic stress exposes the brain cells to high levels of cortisol, which actually causes brain cells to shrink in size. Long-standing stress can cause progressive damage of these brain cells and may even lead to Alzheimer's disease.

How do all of these diseases and conditions develop as a result of stress? To answer that, let's talk about what stress looks like at the physical level. What happens in your body during moments of stress?

> Because of God's tender mercy, the morning light from heaven is about to break upon us, to give light to those who sit in darkness and in the shadow of death, and to guide us to the path of peace.
> —LUKE 1:78–79

UNDERSTANDING STRESS

Dr. Hans Selye is considered by many to be the father of stress research since he was the first to document research related to prolonged release of fight-or-flight hormones into the body. An endocrinologist, Selye initially was attempting in his research to find the next new female hormone. He injected rats with an extract of ovarian tissue and then observed the effects of the hormone. Selye was a somewhat clumsy investigator, however, and would frequently drop the rats after injecting them, chase them around his lab, and use a broom to get them to move from behind a desk or file cabinet. At the end of this experiment, he did autopsies on the rats and found that most had developed ulcers, shrunken thymus glands, and enlarged adrenal glands. He was surprised that the ovarian extract would produce these effects. He decided to perform another experiment with tighter controls.

The second time, instead of using an ovarian extract on all the rats, he injected half of them with saline, a form of salt water. Again, he was sloppy in his handling of the rats, dropping and chasing them as he had the first time. At the end of this experiment he again autopsied the rats and found the same findings—in both groups! He used the phrase "general adaptation syndrome" to describe how the rats had responded to chronic stress. Through these experiments Dr. Selye determined that when stress is maintained long enough, the body undergoes three distinctly different stages. He called these stages:

- The alarm stage
- The resistance stage
- The exhaustion stage

We're going to look closely at these three different stress stages. Take note of your own stress symptoms, and see if you can determine the stage of stress you may be experiencing.

STAGE 1—THE ALARM STAGE

A few years ago my wife, my son, and my nephew went over to a neighbor's house to retrieve a paddleboat they had borrowed. As soon as they got out of the truck, they spotted a huge pit bull on the second-story balcony of the house. As my son, Kyle, began walking toward the lake where the boat was docked, the pit bull jumped off the balcony and began chasing him. Thinking fast, Kyle ran to the dock and jumped into the water. The dog chased him, jumped into the water after him, and began swimming toward him. Kyle took off his sandal and hit the dog on the head every time it lunged at him. Finally the dog became frustrated, turned around, and swam to shore.

My nephew was in the yard watching, and since he had two pit bulls himself, he thought he could befriend this one. "Come here, boy," he called, but the pit bull came charging at him, barking ferociously and foaming at the mouth. Realizing the dog intended to maul him, my nephew went into defense mode, and as the dog charged at him, my nephew hit him as hard has he could with his fist. Even though the hit sounded as loud as the crack of a bat hitting a baseball, it only knocked the huge pit bull back a few steps. The dog shook it off and charged at my nephew again and again.

As my nephew kept hitting the dog and trying to dodge it, he could hear my wife, Mary, about fifty yards away, yelling, "Don't look the dog in his eyes." She had recently seen a documentary on dog attacks, and it had warned never to make eye contact with an angry dog because he sees it as a threat.

The dog finally got hold of my nephew's leg and began tearing at his flesh. Mary screamed loudly, and the dog turned around and headed straight for her. When she saw the pit bull coming at her, she immediately put into practice what the documentary had advised. She turned her back to the dog and folded her arms. As the dog approached, she began slowly turning to avoid eye contact. The pit bull ran in a circle trying to obtain eye contact with Mary, but she just continued to slowly turn away from the dog and was able to avoid eye contact.

Although it felt like hours, a few minutes later animal control arrived and captured the dog. Soon afterward Mary, Kyle, and my nephew came to my office to be treated. Kyle and my nephew were actually laughing and joking as they told me about the ordeal.

You see, Kyle ran and swam and burned off most of his stress hormones. My nephew fought and dodged and burned off most of his stress hormones. But Mary neither ran nor fought but instead slowly turned. You could say she was "stewing in her own stress juices." Kyle and my nephew had perfectly normal blood pressure, heart rates, and other vital signs, but Mary's heart rate was rapid, her fists were clenched, her shoulders were tight and raised up, her neck and back muscles were tense, and she complained of a headache.

Chronic stress causes muscle contraction and pain. Mary was reliving the dog attack and thinking, "What if I, my son, or my nephew had been mauled or killed?" Luckily we went on a cruise the very next day, and she was able to relax, get a massage, laugh, and "unstick" her stuck stress response, thus turning off her stress hormones.

In the case of Mary, Kyle, and my nephew, they first experienced the alarm stage. The alarm stage is the fight-or-flight emergency alarm system that God created in your body for survival. In the case of your ancestors, this protective system would have gone into action when your great-grandfather encountered a bear as he hunted in the woods.

It's similar to a red light and an ear-deafening siren going off in the hypothalamus, an area in the brain. Now the brain is on red alert; therefore, it sends a signal to the pituitary gland to release a hormone that activates the adrenal glands.

Adrenaline (or epinephrine), a hormone that is released from the emergency alert adrenal glands located just above the kidneys, races through the body, sending it into high alert. The brain becomes very focused, eyesight sharpens, and muscles tense as they prepare for fighting or fleeing. Heart rate and blood pressure increase as blood vessels constrict. The bronchial tubes dilate so that you can take in more oxygen. Fuel in the form of fats and sugars are released into the bloodstream. The blood also clots faster.

Primed for the fight

In the story about Mary, Kyle, and my nephew, their hearts were pounding, their breathing was faster and deeper, and their blood sugar rose to supply fuel for their muscles.

This alarm stage of stress sets in motion a release of fats—an emergency fuel supply. Triglycerides, which are fats, are dumped into the bloodstream. These fats as well as sugars fuel the muscles for fighting or fleeing. Blood is shunted away from the stomach and intestines—there's no time for digesting food, and besides, the body needs this extra blood to be pumped to the muscles to enable them to run farther or fight harder.

In this state the digestive tract shuts down or at least functions at a much-diminished capacity. The secretion of saliva slows down as well.

The thyroid is stimulated too, increasing the metabolic rate as it kicks out thyroid hormone. Blood is able to clot faster, which in my family's case could have saved their lives if they had been bleeding as a result of their attack.

By the time Kyle and my nephew got back to my office, their stress reaction had returned to normal. But Mary's stress response had become stuck temporarily as she neither fled nor fought but was reliving the attack and stewing in her own stress juices.

What an incredible creation our bodies are! This amazing alarm system provided what pioneers needed to face the challenges of wagon trains, wild animal attacks, and prairie fires.

Immersed in the amazing tranquility of God's creation, the body would quickly return to a healthy, normally functioning state.

Mental stress vs. physical stress

Rarely does anyone in modern times experience animal attacks, muggings, accidents, or other physical attacks or stressors. The majority of our stress is mental and emotional stress: deadlines at work, financial pressures, mounting debt, traffic jams, relationship stress, and news broadcasts that continually focus on bad news such as crime, unemployment, economic downturns, political unrest, wars, terrorism, etc.

However, *all* forms of stress, whether they are physical,

mental, or emotional, produce the same reactions in your body. The body's stress response creates more than fourteen hundred known physical and chemical reactions, involving more than thirty different hormones and neurotransmitters. God programmed the body this way to help mankind survive all kinds of danger and attacks.

The stress response that a caveman or pioneer would have had during a physical encounter with a wild animal in years past might take place in your body ten, twenty, thirty, or even a hundred times daily due to the mental and emotional stresses of modern life. Today's psychological and emotional stress is far more constant and continuous than an occasional prairie fire or wild animal attack.

Because of this constant nature of modern-day stress, our bodies are not able to dissipate the stress chemicals as our ancestors could. Stress chemicals continuously flood into our systems, preparing our bodies to either fight or flee. But many of us can only fume as we sit stranded in traffic with nothing to do while these chemicals race through our bodies raising our blood pressure, increasing our blood sugar, increasing our cholesterol, increasing our fats, raising cortisol levels, and slowly causing our bones to melt away. Therefore, we end up literally stewing in our own juices.

Our bodies are being bombarded with powerful stress chemicals with no outlet because we are constantly undergoing powerful stress responses for seemingly frivolous reasons. Stress chemicals are being released driving to work, in disagreements with fellow employees, in conflicts with a spouse, dealing with rebellious teenagers, and as we participate in the political and financial turmoil of modern times.

God designed this emergency alarm system to be used to save our lives by fleeing or fighting. Instead, these stress chemicals are being triggered in our bodies hundreds of times a day, and as a result, chronic, degenerative diseases are killing Americans at earlier and earlier ages. The Bible tells us that men's hearts will fail them for fear in the last days. (See Luke 21:26.) This is happening right now!

STAGE 2—THE RESISTANCE STAGE

As we mentioned, the number of individuals visiting doctors' offices for stress-related disorders is at an all-time high. As I see patients, I've noticed that some come when they are suffering only from the alarm stage of stress. But the great majority of stressed-out individuals I see are suffering the later resistance or exhaustion stages of stress. The chances are that if you have been dealing with too much stress for a prolonged time, you may be among that majority.

Let's look at the progression of these dangerous stress levels as they move into the second stage: the resistance stage.

When your body's stress response becomes stimulated more frequently, or if you are experiencing stress overload, anxiety, depression, grief, bitterness, or other negative emotions, you are probably in the resistance stage of stress. This stage can kick in, for example, with an extended time of unemployment, a chronic illness, long-standing marital problems, the grief of having a child on drugs, a long-term financial crisis, or any other negative circumstances that produce an ongoing feeling of anxiety, fear, hopelessness, helplessness, depression, anger, or bitterness.

Usually when your body enters the resistance stage of stress, it continually pumps powerful stress chemicals into your bloodstream, including the highly charged hormones cortisol and adrenaline.

The hypothalamus usually becomes chronically stimulated. It, in turn, stimulates the pituitary gland to release the hormone that activates the adrenal glands. These little glands that sit above the kidneys release cortisol and adrenaline and continually pump them into your body. In stage 2, elevated levels of both cortisol and adrenaline are usually present.

Commander cortisol

Cortisol is a stress hormone that God placed within each of us to help sustain us during a prolonged crisis. During months of disease or other difficult circumstances of protracted stress or illness, this powerful hormone can save your life.

However, when you are continually living and working under significant levels of stress, your risk of developing the illnesses listed in the Bible Cure Health Tip "Physical Results of Excessive Stress" goes up. To understand why, you need to first understand that in a stress response in stage 2, elevated cortisol levels play a major role in many stress-related health conditions.

Diabetes

A prolonged release of cortisol can lead to insulin resistance and elevated blood sugar levels. In the alarm stage these hormones are released, and blood sugar levels become elevated for a very short duration of time. Then, when the crisis is over, they return to normal. But when cortisol levels become chronically elevated, your blood sugar may begin to rise, leading to increased insulin levels and insulin resistance. Over time this may lead to prediabetes and diabetes as insulin receptors become more resistant to insulin.

Triglycerides, which are released into your bloodstream as fuel, may also stay elevated. High levels of triglycerides are associated with heart disease and a fatty liver.

Weight gain

Cortisol is very similar to the drug cortisone. If you have ever taken cortisone, you are aware that it causes you to retain fluid. It also causes your body to gain weight, especially in the belly and torso area. That's why those who are dealing with protracted stress often gain weight—especially belly fat—for seemingly no reason.

Bone loss

Cortisol, much like cortisone, can lead to bone loss. Over the long term, elevation of cortisol may lead to osteopenia and eventually osteoporosis. The medication prednisone, which is a type of cortisone, increases one's risk of bone loss with long-term use. Long-term stress with elevated cortisol levels works very similarly.

Elevated blood pressure

High levels of cortisol for extended periods of time may elevate your blood pressure by robbing your body of vital minerals such as magnesium, potassium, and calcium. Magnesium, potassium, and calcium are extremely important in maintaining normal blood pressure.

You already may be aware of how important these minerals are to maintaining strong, healthy bones. Elevated cortisol levels usually cause the body to retain sodium, which may also raise your blood pressure. In addition, the stress hormone adrenaline constricts your arteries with similar results.

Memory loss

Not only does cortisol steal minerals, but it can also bankrupt your body's supply of essential vitamins and minerals such as the B vitamins, vitamin C, and zinc. B vitamins are really important for maintaining neurotransmitter levels in your brain for stress control.

Excess cortisol may also damage the brain by creating excessive amounts of free radicals. These free radicals may eventually destroy brain cells. Excess cortisol also may impair glucose uptake by brain cells, thus further contributing to memory loss.

Compromised immune system

High cortisol levels over an extended period of time may also weaken or confuse the immune system. Individuals in the resistance stage of stress also are more prone to bacterial and viral infections, candida, and allergies. You may begin to develop allergy symptoms you've never before experienced—sneezing, runny nose, and itchy eyes, as well as food allergies, food sensitivities, and food intolerances…and the list just keeps on going.

Sleep deprivation

Stress also leads to insomnia and sleep disorders. Individuals in the resistance stage, or stage 2, are usually so revved up they often can't sleep well at night. This is usually due to elevated cortisol levels at night. As you can imagine, without rest stress is increased even more. This downward spiral of stage 2 stress can lead to the third and final stage of stress—exhaustion. At this point, you are headed for a crash and burnout.

STAGE 3—EXHAUSTION

As your body reaches stage 3 of stress, your downward spiral of stress ends in exhaustion. All of your organs and body systems have been on heightened alert by elevated stress hormones for so long that they finally throw up the white flag. Completely spent, you may crash and burn. At stage 3 you've usually either run out of gas or are running on fumes—physically, emotionally, mentally, and spiritually. This is a very dangerous point to reach. Your body has given all it has to give, and now it begins to break down.

When you get to the exhaustion stage, your once robust, powerful body that was designed to remain healthy begins to break down, degenerate, and die prematurely. At this final stage of stress, many dramatic changes take place. Let's take a look at some of them.

Immune system depletion

Your immune system that struggled and faltered at stage 2 can now become even more weakened, opening a Pandora's box. The body is more prone to bacterial, viral, parasitic, and fungal infections; allergies; candida; autoimmune diseases; and many other illnesses.

As the immune system becomes increasingly depleted, it leads to worsened allergies, environmental illness, inflammation of joints, aches and pains, a dramatically reduced resistance to infection, severe fatigue, and worsening insomnia. This state of chronic ill health usually comes with emotional and mental fallout. You may become increasingly anxious, irritable, and even more depressed. The exhaustion stage of stress may lead to chronic conditions of depression, anxiety, fatigue, and fibromyalgia.

If this process isn't halted, autoimmune diseases such as lupus, rheumatoid arthritis, thyroiditis, multiple sclerosis, and eventually even cancer can follow.

> For as [a man] thinketh in his heart, so is he.
> —PROVERBS 23:7, KJV

Decreased sexual functioning

Your supply of adrenaline and cortisol that has been elevated for so long eventually gets used up, and your stress hormone levels usually decline. Your bank account is now overdrawn. As a result, in stage 3 you may experience a decrease in sex hormones such as progesterone, testosterone, and estrogen, which usually adversely affects sexual function. This typically leads to decreased sex drive in men and women.

PMS, perimenopause symptoms, and erectile dysfunction

This decrease in sex hormones can have dramatic consequences for both men and women. Progesterone, the raw material for making the stress hormone cortisol, usually has been depleted because of living under prolonged stress. When your progesterone is depleted, you can develop PMS and symptoms of perimenopause, and you may start menopause much earlier than you would otherwise. Chronic stress may cause testosterone levels to plummet in men, causing erectile dysfunction, loss of sex drive, loss of a competitive drive, and loss of a zest for life. They also become grumpy, irritable, and hard to live with. I have seen this even in men in their thirties.

A **BIBLE CURE** *Health Fact*

Are You Exhausted? A Test for Adrenal Exhaustion

If you feel dizzy or lightheaded when you stand up suddenly, it may be an indicator that you are in the exhaustion stage of stress.

A simple screening test for adrenal exhaustion is to have your blood pressure checked while lying down. Rest for five minutes. Then stand up and immediately have your blood pressure checked again. If it drops by ten points, it's very likely that your adrenals are exhausted. Just be sure that you are not dehydrated, because that can produce the same effect.

I test patients' adrenal function by checking salivary cortisol levels at 8:00 a.m., noon, 4:00 p.m., and 8:00 p.m. I also check DHEA sulfate levels. (See Appendix B for more information.)

Weight gain

If you've been gaining weight for seemingly no reason, it may indicate that your body has progressed to the exhaustion stage of the stress response.

The functioning of your thyroid can also be diminished in the exhaustion stage. Remember, during the alarm stage the thyroid responds by increasing the metabolic rate. During stage 3, your adrenals have become exhausted, which may also impair thyroid function. Stress impairs the conversion of T4 (thyroxine) to T3 (triiodothyronine). T3 is a thyroid hormone that is about four times more powerful than T4 and may help with weight loss. Therefore, if you are in stage 3, you may have developed a low-functioning thyroid gland, which often is accompanied by a significant weight gain.

Don't forget that at this stage the neurotransmitters in your brain may be imbalanced as well. It is very common during stage 3 that your serotonin levels may be diminished, which usually causes you to crave sugar, starches, and chocolate. Low serotonin levels may also be associated with depression.

Low blood sugar (hypoglycemia)

Adrenal exhaustion also may cause the blood sugar to drop. Along with low levels of serotonin, dramatic dips in blood sugar levels may also create cravings for sweets, starches, and chocolate.

Because adrenaline and cortisol tend to raise blood sugar, your blood sugar may drop significantly when your reserves of these hormones have been exhausted. You may find yourself needing to eat every couple of hours, or else you feel starved, cranky, and irritable.

With the increased calories, you then tend to gain even more weight as you frequently satisfy your craving for more starches, sugars, and other carbohydrates. You may even start losing muscle mass as you gain weight. Weight is usually gained in the abdomen, the thighs, and the hips.

Very often muscle mass is lost in the arms, legs, and buttocks. What happens to many men is that much of their weight shifts downward. Many get "furniture disease," where their chest shifts down to their "drawers." You've seen men with this disease; they walk around with big bellies that look about nine months pregnant and with skinny little arms and legs and flat buttocks. Many such individuals are suffering from the adrenal exhaustion stage of stress. Unaware of this, they may blame their Humpty-Dumpty look on aging.

Loss of muscle mass

Cortisol is the only hormone that increases with aging. It is a catabolic hormone that causes one to lose muscle mass, especially in the larger muscle groups of the thighs, buttocks, back, and shoulders. Also in the exhaustion stage of stress many are simply too tired to exercise to maintain muscle mass. The greater the muscle loss, the lower the metabolic rate, making one more susceptible to weight gain.

Digestive problems

As symptoms of stage 3 stress continue to spiral downward, your stomach and pancreas can be affected as well. The stomach can begin producing either too much or too little acid. Either of these extremes is harmful and can lead to heartburn, bloating, gas, and symptoms of reflux. Too little acid may impair digestion. You may also produce inadequate amounts of pancreatic enzymes.

Inadequate amounts of pancreatic enzymes and hydrochloric acid typically cause poor fat, carbohydrate, and protein digestion and absorption. This can also cause you to lose muscle mass while still gaining fat.

Memory loss

Do you find yourself looking into the face of someone whose name you know but are not able to pull up the information? Prolonged stress impacts your ability to remember things.

The continual pumping of cortisol into our bodies actually damages and may destroy brain cells. It is like pouring acid on your brain. This degenerative process can eventually lead to memory loss and possibly even Alzheimer's disease. Nevertheless, even a moderate state of memory loss can usually be completely turned around if it's caught in time.

Autoimmune disease

A final stop of this destructive downhill fall may be autoimmune disease. At this point, instead of the body protecting itself as it has been working very hard to do through stage 1 and stage 2, it may actually begin attacking itself. That's what autoimmune diseases are all about.

When stress is not dealt with or treated, it can become a violent aggressor, causing your body to damage itself through autoimmune diseases such as lupus, rheumatoid arthritis, thyroiditis, Hashimoto's thyroiditis, multiple sclerosis, type 1 diabetes, and many more. Your body may have become so run-down that you have opened a door to disaster.

> I am leaving you with a gift—peace of mind and heart. And the peace I give is a gift the world cannot give. So don't be troubled or afraid.
>
> —JOHN 14:27

THERE'S HOPE FOR YOU!

Don't be alarmed if you see yourself in this destructive downward spiral of stress and disease. There is hope for you. Even if your world feels as if it is filled with stress, you have reason to be extremely encouraged.

Jesus Christ said, "In the world ye shall have tribulation: but be of good cheer; I have overcome the world" (John 16:33, KJV).

Jesus Christ has the answer for the stressful lives that so many of us feel forced to live.

As you continue to read through this book on stress, you will become increasingly aware that God's plan for you is good health—body, mind, and spirit. Better yet, He holds the power over every force in the universe—even your stress. He has answers to your every question and peace for your every fear.

You will conquer stress; it will not conquer you. With God's help, you cannot lose. So, read on and get ready to win the battle!

> But when the Holy Spirit produces this kind of fruit in our lives: love, joy, peace, patience, kindness, goodness, faithfulness, gentleness, and self-control.
> —Galatians 5:22–23

A **BIBLE CURE** Prayer for You

Dear Lord Jesus, I thank You that You overcame the entire world through Your death on the cross. Your power is greater than any force in the entire universe—even stress. In fact, You hold the universe. Thank You for putting this book in my hands to show me the way to conquer stress and its dangerous effects in my life. Amen.

A **BIBLE** **CURE** *Prescription*

What are your stress-related symptoms?

_____

_____

_____

_____

What level of stress do you believe you may be experiencing? Why?

_____

_____

_____

_____

In your own words, thank God for His help in overcoming the dangerous downward spiral of stress.

_____

_____

_____

_____

Chapter 2

SUPPLEMENT STRATEGIES FOR COPING WITH STRESS

O UR STRESSFUL LIFESTYLES really can feel overwhelming at times. If stress has ever left you feeling defeated and depleted, the Bible has the answer. You see, stress is nothing new. David wrote in the Psalms, "When my heart is overwhelmed: lead me to the rock that is higher than I" (Ps. 61:2, KJV).

In a demanding, turbulent world, it's comforting to remember that Christ is greater than your greatest problem. His tender love is a rock you can stand upon no matter how much the world shakes around you.

You can go to God when you feel overwhelmed and stressed. But what do we do instead? Many of us go to the refrigerator seeking a little "comfort" food to get us through the current round of stress. A slice of pie or a batch of chocolate chip cookies does nothing to reduce your stress. As a matter of fact, as we have seen, sugar can be harmful to an already stressed-out body. It gives a momentary lift, but you've actually further taxed your body and have not dealt with the roots of your stress.

To recover from the sense of burnout, exhaustion, and nervous tension of stress, you are going to need to deal with the physical roots that are affecting your emotions and your sense of well-being.

You now realize that stress has wreaked havoc on your physical body and your emotions. Gaining control over stress and its unpleasant side effects will involve bringing your physical body back to a healthier state. This can be accomplished through supplements and nutrition.

Stress and high cortisol levels also may deplete certain nutrients in the body. People who are under excessive stress nearly always need to have an increase in the B vitamins (especially pantothenic acid, B_5), vitamin C, magnesium, zinc, copper, chromium, selenium, and vitamin E.

THE B VITAMINS: KEY TO STRESS RELIEF

The B vitamins (thiamin, riboflavin, niacin, pantothenic acid, folic acid, vitamin B_6, and vitamin B_{12}) are often called the "stress-relief vitamins." The B-vitamin family provides the greatest benefit when supplemented together, such as a balanced B complex. Some B vitamins actually require other B vitamins for activation. The B vitamins are especially important for elderly individuals since B vitamins are not absorbed as well as a person ages. The B vitamins are associated primarily with brain and nervous system function.

Pantothenic acid (B_5)

Pantothenic acid is known as the "antistress" vitamin because it plays such a vital role in the production of adrenal hormones. A deficiency of pantothenic acid leads to a decreased resistance to stress.[1] Pantothenic acid provides critical support for the adrenal glands as it responds to stress, and adequate supplementation is very important for the health of adrenal glands in most people. I believe vitamin B_5 is the most important B vitamin for restoring and maintaining adrenal function. I typically place patients with adrenal fatigue on 500 mg, two times a day.

Pantothenic acid can be found in salmon, yeast, vegetables, dairy, eggs, grains, and meat.

Vitamin B_6

Vitamin B_6 is vital for the utilization of amino acids (which are the building blocks for proteins). A vitamin B_6 deficiency is often marked by depression, irritability, nervousness, muscle weakness, dermatitis, slow learning, numbness, and cramping in the extremities. B_6 is required by the nervous system and is needed for normal brain function. It is needed to produce dopamine, serotonin, and GABA (gamma-amino butyric acid). These are very important neurotransmitters for promoting feelings of well-being, relaxation, and calmness.

Vitamin B_6 is especially important for women using oral contraceptives (birth control pills) and experiencing bouts of depression, irritability, moodiness, fatigue, and decreased sex drive. Many of these symptoms can be reversed with B_6 supplementation.[2] Food sources for B_6 include lentils, lima beans, soybeans, sunflower seeds, bananas, avocados, buckwheat, and brewer's yeast.

Vitamin B_{12}

A vitamin B_{12} deficiency has been related to peripheral neuropathy, anemia, paresthesias, demyelination of the dorsal columns and corticospinal tract of the spinal cord, depression, dementia, and heart disease. A deficiency has also been associated with low energy, poor memory, problems in thinking, low stomach acid, and elevated homocysteine levels.[3]

A study conducted at Tufts University found that nearly 40 percent of those studied had a B_{12} blood level in "low normal" range, which is where neurological symptoms begin to occur. The individuals between the ages of twenty-six and forty-nine were discovered to have the same high risk for B_{12} deficiency as those over the age of sixty-five.[4]

Vitamin B_{12} is also important for maintaining the myelin sheaths that cover and protect nerve endings. Subclinical or borderline B_{12} deficiency is rather common, especially among the elderly.[5]

We know from nutrition-related research that much of vitamins B_6, B_{12}, and folic acid are destroyed in the processing and refining of foods. With so many Americans hooked on highly processed foods, fast foods, and foods that contain high amounts of sugar, it is probable that countless American adults are suffering from borderline or frank deficiency in these B vitamins. This may be one reason cardiovascular disease is escalating at such a great rate and why stress-related diseases are so rampant. After all, B-complex vitamins are known as the stress-relief vitamins.

VITAMIN C: A KEY ANTISTRESS ANTIOXIDANT

Vitamin C is an extremely important vitamin and antioxidant in the battle against stress. It is more concentrated in the adrenal glands than almost anywhere else in the body.[6] The adrenal glands use more vitamin C per gram of tissue weight than any other organ or tissue in the body.

A number of research studies have confirmed that vitamin C has a significant ability to decrease stress. An example is a study at the University of Alabama that concluded vitamin C supplementation significantly decreased stress hormone levels in laboratory rats. The vitamin C also decreased other typical indicators of physical and emotional stress, such as enlargement of the adrenal glands and reduction in size of the thymus and spleen.[7]

Vitamin C is an antioxidant, and as such, it has indirect benefits related to stress. As we have noted previously, chronic stress raises both cortisol and adrenaline in the body. These hormones increase free-radical production, which creates "oxidative stress."

Antioxidants are compounds that help protect the cells from free-radical damage. They are able to disarm free radicals.

Antioxidants work synergistically, or as a "team," in the body. For example, vitamin C helps to restore vitamin E to its full potency. Other water-soluble antioxidants that help protect the cells from free-radical damage are pine bark extract, grape seed extract, green tea extract, quercetin, and most phytonutrients. (Phytonutrients are found in fruits and vegetables and are also readily available in supplement form.)

The current RDI (reference daily intake) for vitamin C is 75–90 mg a day to prevent disease. I recommend 500–3,000 mg a day for optimal daily intake. As a water-soluble vitamin, any vitamin C that is consumed and isn't needed by the body will be flushed out through the bloodstream and kidneys.

Medications such as aspirin and oral contraceptives deplete vitamin C in the body. People who develop kidney stones or are on numerous medications should consult their physician about taking additional vitamin C.

GLUTATHIONE: THE MOTHER OF ALL ANTIOXIDANTS

Glutathione is an important antioxidant that functions as a detoxifier of the body, neutralizing toxins and heavy metals as well as quenching free radicals. It helps maintain your body's energy, protects the mitochondria (where ATP, or energy, is produced), improves your immune system function, and helps support the adrenal glands.

Glutathione is produced in your body and recycled by your body all the time—except when the toxic load becomes too great. Chronic stress may lead to excessive oxidative stress in your body, causing your glutathione levels to drop and compromising your body's protection against free radicals, infections, and illnesses. It becomes harder for your body to get rid of the toxins as well. This creates a vicious cycle of chronic illness.

In a recent *Huffington Post* article, Mark Hyman, MD, wrote of his discovery that people with nearly every chronic illness are depleted in glutathione and boosting their intracellular glutathione levels may help their condition improve.[8] There are different ways to raise and support your glutathione levels:

- Supplement with NAC (N-acetyl cysteine). NAC has been proven to boost glutathione levels in the body. (See Appendix B.)

- Supplement with a form of whey protein that contains cysteine, which is a precursor to glutathione. This means your body makes glutathione from cysteine. (See Appendix B.)

- Find a doctor who can administer a glutathione IV. (See Appendix B.)
- Take a glutathione-boosting supplement. (See Appendix B.)

Antistress Benefit From Magnesium

Magnesium is involved in the activation of more than three hundred different enzymes in the body. It is vital to health.

Magnesium is one of the few essential nutrients for which deficiencies are fairly common. One survey showed that 75 percent of Americans did not take in the daily recommended amount of magnesium.[9]

Approximately 99 percent of magnesium in sugar cane is lost when the cane is refined to white sugar, and between 80 and 96 percent of magnesium in wheat is removed when it is refined to white flour.[10]

When cortisol and adrenaline levels are elevated, there is also an increase of urinary excretion of magnesium. This indicates that in times of stress, our bodies have an increased need for magnesium.

The characteristic signs and symptoms of magnesium deficiency include muscle cramps, muscle spasms, hyperventilation, and weakness. Low levels of magnesium in the diet increase a person's risk for developing a wide variety of diseases and ailments, including high blood pressure, heart disease, insomnia, kidney stones, multiple sclerosis, headaches, and menstrual cramps.

I have found in my medical practice that a person may register a "normal" blood serum magnesium level but may actually have a deficit in intracellular magnesium. Therefore I commonly check RBC magnesium levels, which is a more reliable test for magnesium in the body.

Good dietary sources of magnesium include wheat bran, wheat germ, nuts, blackstrap molasses, legumes, and whole grains. The dietary recommendation for magnesium is 400–420 mg a day for men and 310–320 mg a day for women. I commonly recommend 200 mg of magnesium two times a day.

Magnesium, as well as other minerals, is necessary for sustaining bone density and cellular metabolism related to digestion, adrenal function, and liver function.

SUPPLEMENT STRATEGIES FOR THE STRESSED OUT

Let's take a look at some supplement solutions that will dramatically impact the way you feel both physically and emotionally.

Phosphatidylserine

Phosphatidylserine (PS) is an essential component in every cell membrane in the body. It is found in high concentrations in the brain, and it may help prevent a decline in mental function. One study has shown benefits from PS supplements for early Alzheimer's disease patients—in the study, PS supplements were given for three to twelve weeks at a dose of 300 mg per day.[11] PS has also been shown to buffer the overproduction of cortisol, especially after intense exercise. In one study, healthy

European men were given 800 mg of PS a day for ten days prior to cycling to the "near exhaustion" point. They were found to have a 30 percent decrease in cortisol production even after strenuous exercise compared to those who did not receive the PS supplements.[12] Athletes may benefit from taking up to 800 mg a day either prior to training or immediately following training.

I have found that a significant number of patients with adrenal fatigue or low adrenal function have elevated nighttime cortisol levels, which aggravates insomnia. I usually start them on 200 mg of PS in the evening and gradually increase the dose until nighttime cortisol levels are normal.

The average dose of PS is 100 mg in capsule form, and compared to many supplements, PS is quite expensive. Those who are undergoing significant physical stress—such as competitive weight lifters, marathon runners, and others who have elevated nighttime cortisol levels—may find the cost well worth the results. If salivary cortisol levels are elevated in the evening, you may benefit from taking 100–800 mg in the evening or at bedtime.

ADAPTOGENS

An adaptogen is a substance that will help the body adapt to stress by balancing the adrenal gland's response to stress. The end result is that cortisol levels will be neither too high nor too low but will be balanced. Russian scientist Dr. Nicolai Lazarev first used the term *adaptogen* in 1947. The "father of adaptogens," however, is considered to be Dr. Israel Brekhman, who worked at the Far East Science Center of the USSR as head of the Department of Physiology and Pharmacology. He holds forty patents related to the discovery of adaptogenic herbs and applications. Dr. Brekhman describes adaptogens as having these qualities:

1. Completely nontoxic to the human body—with no harmful or negative effects no matter what amount or how long they are used

2. Helpful to the body's mental and physical performance while providing resistance to stressful insults at the cellular level

3. Balance and normalize the body's systems, leading to homeostasis and health

Rhodiola

Rhodiola rosea is also known as "golden root" or "Arctic root." This herb is native to the mountainous regions of Asia, parts of Europe, and the Arctic. Rhodiola is an adaptogen that is said to stimulate the nervous system, decrease depression, eliminate fatigue, increase work performance, enhance immunity, increase exercise capacity, increase memorization skills, and prevent high-altitude sickness. Researchers speculate that rhodiola works by influencing key central nervous system neurotransmitters, including dopamine and serotonin.

I recommend a product that uses a standardization of 2 to 3 percent rosavin, which is the active ingredient of rhodiola used in clinical studies. The common dose is 200–600 mg three times a day.

Ginseng

Ginseng is another adaptogen that may help the body adapt to both physical and psychological stress in both stage 2 and stage 3 stress response. A number of different products are available under the general umbrella of ginseng. Know the ginseng you are considering!

Korean ginseng

Korean ginseng, also called *Panax*, which is the Greek word for "cure-all," has long been used in Chinese medicine. A quality ginseng product should have at least 25 mg of ginsenoside, calculated as ginsenoside Rg1. The standard dose for a Panax ginseng extract that contains 14 percent saponins would be 200 mg. Ginseng is typically taken one to three times a day, and the usual regimen is three weeks on and two weeks off.

Siberian ginseng

Siberian ginseng (SG) has been shown to provide many of the benefits of caffeine but without the post-caffeine "letdown." It seems to improve the use of oxygen in exercising muscle tissues, which means a person might exercise longer and recover more quickly from aerobic exercise. Standardized extracts are generally recommended in doses of 300–400 mg a day. It should be taken continuously for six to eight weeks, followed by a one- to two-week break. Siberian ginseng is available in many forms, including tablets, capsules, extracts, teas, chewing gum, and drinks.

Ashwagandha

The root of the ashwagandha plant is known as "Indian ginseng," and its use can be traced back three thousand years.

The Indian *Materia Medica* recommends using it for impotence, general debility, brain fatigue, low sperm count, nervous exhaustion, as an aphrodisiac, and in any case in which vigor must be restored. Its chemical compounds are similar to those found in ginseng, but it has been shown to be superior in relieving stress when compared to Chinese ginseng. The typical dosage of ashwagandha is 3–6 grams per day.

Magnolia bark

Magnolia bark, *magnolia officinalis*, is a traditional Chinese medicine that has been used for thousands of years to help with low energy, emotional distress, digestive problems, cough, diarrhea, and asthma. Magnolia bark comes from the stem, root, or branch of the magnolia tree. It is known in Chinese medicine as *Hou Po*. Modern research has focused on magnolia for its sedative and muscle relaxant properties. Magnolia does not cause motor impairment, physical dependency, loss of coordination, or memory loss—all of which are potential side effects from typical antianxiety agents such as benzodiazepines. Nevertheless, magnolia has a sedative and relaxing effect. In a recent study, mice were treated with magnolia and diazepam before going through a maze. The magnolia group was more relaxed and finished without any loss of motor activity or muscle tone. The diazepam group had side effects that included drowsiness, disruptive learning and memory, and withdrawal symptoms.[13]

In summary, magnolia extract has the potential to decrease stress, create a calming effect for the nerves, and make a person sleepy.

Magnolia also has strong antioxidant properties. Numerous

studies have revealed that magnolia extract protects mitochondria from free-radical damage in the liver, heart, and brain.[14]

Some research has found that magnolia extract is even more potent than vitamin E in preventing lipid peroxidation, which is a contributor to heart disease and atherosclerosis.[15]

AMINO ACIDS

Chronic stress interferes with neurotransmitters. If stress persists too long, there will eventually occur a lowering of serotonin, which is a neurotransmitter. Low serotonin levels may be associated with impatience, aggression, irritability, and food cravings—all of which are readily associated with being "stressed out." Low serotonin levels in the brain have also been associated with depression, anxiety, obesity, PMS, violent behavior, suicide, alcoholism, compulsive gambling, insomnia, carbohydrate craving, seasonal affective disorder, and migraine headaches. In contrast, adequate brain serotonin levels are associated with feelings of calmness, well-being, security, confidence, concentration, and relaxation. I recommend targeted amino acid therapy (TAAP) to correct neurotransmitter imbalances, and I commonly recommend the following two substances in my practice.

5-HTP

The body manufactures serotonin from the essential amino acid L-tryptophan. This amino acid is converted into 5-hydroxytryptophan (5-HTP). Supplementation with 5-HTP has been shown to raise brain serotonin levels. One study in Europe found 5-HTP to be more effective than medications such as Prozac, and it was found to cause fewer side effects.[16]

The usual dose of 5-HTP is 150–300 mg a day in divided dosages. I typically start patients on 50 mg, three times a day, or 100 mg at bedtime, and then adjust the dose if needed. Individuals who are taking prescription antidepressants, herbal supplements for depression, or weight-loss medications should not combine these with 5-HTP supplements without consulting a physician first.

L-theanine

L-theanine is another amino acid and is commonly found in green tea. L-theanine was initially discovered in 1950 and was approved as a food additive by the Japanese minister of health and welfare in 1964. Only 1 to 2 percent of the dry weight of tea leaves consists of L-theanine. Because of this, a patented enzymatic process was developed in Japan to synthesize 100 percent pure L-theanine. This product has been shown to decrease stress, promote relaxation, calm nervousness, and decrease restlessness. It is non-sedating and promotes concentration in students. I have used this supplement widely and with significant success in treating stressed-out adults and children with ADHD.

L-theanine is able to cross the blood-brain barrier, and it supports the activity of certain neurotransmitters in the brain. L-theanine does not cause daytime drowsiness and is an excellent alternative for benzodiazepines, which are found in many antianxiety medications.

I recommend this substance commonly in my practice. A person can take 100–300 mg a day or more of L-theanine supplements, or consume three to four cups of green tea a day. Be aware, however, that decaffeinated green tea contains little to no L-theanine since the majority of L-theanine is lost during the decaffeination process.

> May God our Father give you grace and peace.
> —COLOSSIANS 1:2

A **BIBLE CURE** *Health Fact*
Adrenal Glandular Supplements

Glandular therapy has been used for thousands of years, all the way back to ancient Egypt. Today, products like Armour Thyroid are still quite popular in treating patients with hypothyroidism (low thyroid function). Adrenal glandular supplements contain protomorphogens or extracts of tissues from the adrenal glands of pigs or cattle. These can be taken orally to support human adrenal function. Glandular substances in pigs and cattle have an "adrenal mix" close to that of the human adrenal glands. Some doctors of natural medicine have used adrenal glandular supplements with their patients for decades and report very positive results.

When a person is in the resistance stage of stress, I typically recommend a few supplements to help them cope with stress and to support their adrenal glands so that they do not go into the exhaustion stage. I usually recommend an adrenal glandular supplement. (See Appendix B.) I also recommend a higher dose of pantothenic acid to support adrenal function. These patients typically benefit from vitamin B complex as well as a multivitamin. I also usually recommend an adaptogen or cordyceps to help them cope with stress. (See Appendix B.) It's also very important for these individuals to get adequate sleep, usually eight hours of sleep per night. I perform a neuroscience adrenal panel to check cortisol levels, DHEA levels, and neurotransmitter levels. I can then adjust their nutrition program accordingly and repeat the test in a few months to ensure that they are responding appropriately. If nighttime cortisol levels are elevated, I usually place them on phosphatidylserine.

A BIBLE CURE Health Fact

The Benefits of Cordyceps Sinensis

Cordyceps sinensis is a fungus with medicinal properties, sometimes called a "medicinal mushroom." It is said to boost the immune system by activating natural killer cells that destroy free radicals in the body. It also appears to reduce fatigue and increase energy levels by increasing the amount of oxygen in the blood and tissues. Because of these benefits it is an extremely helpful supplement for addressing adrenal fatigue.

To unstick the stuck stress response, you must practice the stress-reduction strategies I discuss in my books *Stress Less* and *The Seven Pillars of Health*, especially getting ten belly laughs a day, practicing gratitude, and forgiveness.

If someone is in the exhaustion stage, then they definitely need to have their cortisol levels and DHEA levels checked. I do this by checking salivary hormones and again by performing the neuroscience adrenal panel. I usually find low cortisol levels as well as low DHEA levels.

Patients in the exhaustion stage need the same supplements I recommend for the resistance stage as well as pregnenolone. Pregnenolone is a hormone that is used to make DHEA in the body and also helps protect the brain from the damaging effects of stress. I have found that DHEA lyposomal cream is a superior delivery system for DHEA and delivers adequate amounts of DHEA throughout the day and night. I recommend three pumps for women and five pumps for men, once or twice a day. Apply it to the full length of one arm and rub it in. (See Appendix B.) I also recommend pregnenolone lyposomal cream in the same dosage (three pumps for women and five pumps for men, once or twice a day; see Appendix B). Patients with severe adrenal fatigue may occasionally need bioidentical cortisol as well as stronger adrenal rebuilders. A knowledgeable physician can prescribe bioidentical cortisol. (See Appendix B.)

Finally, I place most patients in the exhaustion stage on the Myers IV, which provides B vitamins, magnesium, vitamin C, and other nutrients. I recommend the Myers IV once a week for eight weeks, then once every two weeks, and so on. For more information on the Myers IV, see Appendix B.

I also recommend supplements that fuel the mitochondria, which help increase ATP and thereby increase your energy levels. (See Appendix B.) Find out about other herbs, supplements, adaptogens, and amino acids that may also be effective for relieving stress and insomnia by referring to *The New Bible Cure for Depression and Anxiety* and *The New Bible Cure for Sleep Disorders*.

A **BIBLE CURE** *Health Fact*
The Benefits of Pregnenolone

Pregnenolone, discovered in the 1940s, is a natural hormone your body manufactures from cholesterol, and it supports adrenal function. It is sometimes called the "grandmother hormone" because it is a precursor to other hormones made by the body, including DHEA (the "mother" hormone), progesterone, testosterone, estrogen, and cortisol. Pregnenolone counters the damage that can be caused by cortisol when you are under prolonged stress, and it helps modulate the transmission of messages from neuron to neuron. In other words, it helps you to think more quickly, understand and remember things more easily, and speak with greater clarity. For more information on pregnenolone and adrenal fatigue, refer to my book *Stress Less*.

> Let this mind be in you, which was also in Christ Jesus.
> —PHILIPPIANS 2:5, KJV

IN CONCLUSION

You don't have to let stress rob you of your strength, energy, vitality, happiness, and joy. You can take back your health by rebuilding your body through powerful supplements. You will feel refreshed, restored, and rejuvenated in no time.

A **BIBLE CURE** *Prayer for You*

*Dear Lord, thank You for providing natural solutions to
restore my health. Grant me the wisdom I need to select
the proper supplements. I thank You for restoring my joy,
energy, happiness, and peace. In Jesus's name, amen.*

A **BIBLE CURE** *Prescription*

List the supplements you are planning to take to help
your body combat stress.

_____

_____

_____

Write a prayer thanking God for your complete recovery from the
negative effects of stress in your life.

_____

_____

_____

Chapter 3

EXERCISE STRATEGIES FOR COPING WITH STRESS

G OD WANTS TO bless you with the peaceful joy of a stress-free life. As a matter of fact, God promises to strengthen your body and to give peace to your mind and soul. The Bible says, "The LORD will give strength to His people; the LORD will bless His people with peace" (Ps. 29:11, NKJV).

A powerful strategy for conquering stress is exercise. Exercise provides an extremely beneficial avenue for releasing pent-up stress and negative emotions. Instead of allowing stress to tear down your body, you can actually use exercise to relieve stress.

A good workout can dissipate stress and leave you feeling great. My son, Kyle, and I coauthored a book called *Get Fit and Live!* that provides you with demonstrations of several workout routines along with tons of information about the benefits and importance of exercise. Let's look at some exercises you can do to conquer stress so that it never conquers you, including some relaxation exercises that will help you to unwind.

THREE-MINUTE RELAXATION ROUTINE

This relaxation routine takes only three minutes, but it can be a lifesaver in a tense situation.

1. Concentrate on relaxing using a cue word or phrase, such as *God's peace* or *God's love.* Listen to your own breathing, and take in one deep breath and hold it in.

2. While you are holding your breath, tense up a group of muscles, such as the muscles in your face, legs, or arms.

3. As you release the breath, relax the tense muscle group. Feel all your tension slip away. Drop your shoulders down and rotate them in a circle.

4. Repeat.

You can do this relaxation exercise while you're at work or at home. Learning to relax takes practice. Relaxation training reduces anxiety and stress, and it decreases the risk of heart disease and high blood pressure.[1]

PROGRESSIVE MUSCLE RELAXATION

In this relaxation exercise you must tighten each muscle group in your body, hold it for five seconds, and then gradually release the muscles and relax them for ten to fifteen seconds. Relaxing your entire body through this technique will take about twenty minutes.

1. Sit or lie down quietly in a comfortable position away from noise or distractions.

2. Scan your body to identify areas of stress or tension.

3. Begin to tense and tighten your muscles in each of the following muscle groups, beginning at your head. Tense each body part for five seconds, and then slowly release the tension as you focus on the body part. This needs to be repeated twice for each muscle group. As you learn to slowly release the tension in your muscles, you will actually be teaching your body how to relax.

- Forehead and top of head—raise eyebrows
- Jaw—clench teeth
- Neck—pull chin forward onto your chest
- Shoulders and trapezoid muscles—lift shoulders
- Back—pull back shoulder blades
- Arms—flex biceps
- Abdomen—tighten abdomen
- Buttocks—squeeze and tighten buttocks
- Thighs—flex thighs
- Calves—flex and point toes up or down[2]

A **BIBLE CURE** *Health Tip*
Melt Away Stress

Essential oils can be added directly to your bath water. Here's how:

- Add 5–10 drops of essential oils to hot water while filling your bath.
- Do not combine essential oils with other bath oils or soap.
- Make sure to soak in the tub for at least twenty minutes to get the aromatic benefits.

You can find essential oils at health food stores. The following essential oils have properties that are especially beneficial.

- **Lavender.** At first this oil may pep you up a little. But as you soak for a few minutes, you'll find that it calms you. It relieves nervous tension, depression, and insomnia.
- **Geranium.** Combine a couple drops of this with lavender. It has a calming effect.
- **Rosemary.** This one helps circulation. Use it alone or with lavender to relieve depression.
- **Baking soda or Epsom salts.** A hot bath in baking soda can do wonders for relaxing your muscles. Scoop a handful of baking soda or 1–2 cups of Epsom salts into very hot bath water and relax.

GET HOOKED ON REGULAR EXERCISE

Regular aerobic exercise doesn't have to be a chore. As a matter of fact, it can be a lot of fun. Instead of always getting together with your friends for lunch or dessert, why not try meeting your friends for a walk or game of tennis?

Brisk walking or bicycling are great ways to get in shape and release stress. What about joining a square dancing club or taking ballroom dancing lessons? I guarantee you'll wonder why you didn't try it sooner.

A **BIBLE CURE** *Health Tip*
A Simple Walking Program

(NOTE: Each column indicates the number of minutes to walk. Complete three exercise sessions each week. If you find a particular week's pattern tiring, repeat it before going on to the next pattern. You do not have to complete the walking program in twelve weeks.)

Week	Walk	Walk Briskly	Walk	Total Minutes Walked
1	5	5	5	15
2	5	7	5	17
3	5	9	5	19
4	5	11	5	21
5	5	13	5	23
6	5	15	5	25
7	5	18	5	28
8	5	20	5	30
9	5	23	5	33
10	5	26	5	36
11	5	28	5	38
12	5	30	5	40

Week 13 and thereafter: Check your pulse periodically to see if you are exercising within your target heart rate zone. As you get more in shape, try exercising more within the upper range of your target zone.

Gradually increase your brisk walking time from thirty to forty-five minutes, four or five times a week. Remember that your goal is to get the benefits you are seeking and enjoy your activity.

Regular exercise improves heart health, lung function, circulation, and blood pressure. It reduces fat and lowers cholesterol. Regular exercise relaxes your muscles, reduces stress, and decreases fatigue. As you exercise, your body also releases endorphins, which are natural antidepressants and pain relievers that make you feel better.

So, to relieve your stress, boost your self-image, build your confidence, and increase your energy, determine to start exercising twenty minutes a day at least three days per week, but work up to five days a week.

A BIBLE CURE Health Tip
Your Target Heart Rate Zone

Use the following formula to determine your target heart rate zone while exercising. Once you have determined your desired range, stay within it.

220 minus [your age] = _____

x .65 = _____

[This is your minimum target heart rate.]

220 minus [your age] = _____

x .80 = _____

[This is your maximum target heart.]

This example may help: To calculate the target heart zone for a forty-year-old, subtract the age (40) from 220 (220- 40=180). Multiply 180 by .65, which equals 117. Then multiply 180 by .80, which equals 144. The target heart rate zone is 117–144 beats per minute for a forty-year-old.

A word of caution: If you feel you are in the exhaustion stage of stress, wait a few months until you build up your body with adequate nutrition and rest before getting into an aerobic exercise program, and only exercise three days a week with a day off in between.

> For thus saith the Lord, Behold, I will extend peace to her like a river.
>
> —Isaiah 66:12, kjv

In Conclusion

The apostle Paul said, "But I discipline my body and bring it into subjection, lest, when I have preached to others, I myself should become disqualified" (1 Cor. 9:27, nkjv). Paul's life was filled with stressful situations. Still, he took charge over his body through discipline. In that way he avoided being defeated by the effects of stress.

What about you? Why not choose to conquer stress and its devastating effects on your body? Why not make up your mind right now to include regular exercise in your lifestyle choices? Exercise can make a stressful period of life more bearable. It can make a lifestyle of stress endurable. Exercise can give you the strength you need to go the distance.

A **BIBLE CURE** *Prayer for You*

Dear Lord, give me the discipline and motivation I need
to invest faithfully in a regular program of exercise to
help me manage stress. Thank You for Your promise
to strengthen me—body, mind, and spirit. Amen.

A **BIBLE CURE** *Prescription*

Write out your plan for a regular exercise program that
includes stress-management techniques.

_____

_____

_____

_____

Write a prayer in your own words asking God for His help to keep
you at it.

_____

_____

_____

_____

Chapter 4

MENTAL STRATEGIES FOR COPING WITH STRESS

B ELIEVE IT OR not, you can live a life that is free of the negative effects of stress. God actually promises a way to have a peaceful, happy mind no matter how stressful your circumstances. The prophet declared to God, "You will keep him in perfect peace, whose mind is stayed on You, because he trusts in You" (Isa. 26:3, NKJV).

The Bible provides a strategy for living free from the negative effects associated with stress. You can live in God's wonderful peace every day of your life no matter what disappointments you face, what pressures you must endure, and no matter how many difficult, stressful circumstances surround your life.

It almost sounds too good to be true, but it's not. Let's take a look at some strategies from the Bible that promise peace—no matter what!

RENEWING YOUR MIND

We have mentioned that not everyone experiences the same stress reactions to the same life events. For one person, speaking in front of a large group feels like a fun challenge, but it makes another individual a nervous wreck. If one person's relaxation is another person's stress, then circumstances are not the sole cause of stress. Your individual perception of the events in your life plays a vital role in your experience of stress as well.

Therefore, a powerful strategy for conquering stress is to deal with the roots of stress in your own life by beginning to change your own perceptions and reactions to circumstances. This powerful strategy is taken directly from the Bible. The apostle Paul declared:

> Don't copy the behavior and customs of this world, but let God transform you into a new person by changing the way you think. Then you will know God's will for you, which is good and pleasing and perfect.
>
> —ROMANS 12:2

With God's help, we can develop new, less stressful ways of thinking. Doing so, in fact, is a command from God's Word. It says, "Be renewed in the spirit of your mind" (Eph. 4:23, NKJV).

Renewing the mind is nothing more than breaking the thought patterns and ways of thinking and perceiving life's circumstances that cause us stress. I call these stressful patterns "stinking thinking." Let's take a look at some successful strategies for renewing the mind by breaking the power of stressful stinking thinking.

PRACTICING MINDFULNESS

The concept of mindfulness, studied and explained best by Herbert Benson, MD, is the practice of learning to pay attention to what is happening to you from moment to moment. To be mindful, according to Benson, you must slow down, do one activity at a time, and bring your full awareness to both the activity at hand and to your inner experience of it.[1] Mindfulness provides a potentially powerful antidote to the common causes of daily stress.

Benson's definition of mindfulness reminds me of the words of Jesus: "Therefore do not worry about tomorrow, for tomorrow will worry about its own things. Sufficient for the day is its own trouble" (Matt. 6:34, NKJV). Jesus taught us to be mindful of the present, not of the future. The apostle Paul likewise taught us to forget "those things which are behind," meaning the past (Phil. 3:13). Mindfulness means letting go of any thought that is unrelated to the present moment and finding something to enjoy in the present moment.

But most people do not live in the present moment. They are wishing for a different moment—either past or future. They go through the motions required to function in the present moment, but they are thinking things like "I'll be happy when..."

- "I get a bigger home."
- "I get that promotion."
- "My kids are out of school."
- "I pay off these bills."
- "I get a new car."
- "I lose twenty pounds."

Mindfulness works differently. It trains your mind to let go of any thought that is unrelated to the present moment and to find something to enjoy in the present—continually. When you walk or drive, pay attention to the beautiful scenery, the chirping of the birds and crickets, and the feel of the warm sunshine or the chill in the air. Focus on the way your body feels as you go through routine motions of driving, opening the door, walking to your destination. During work breaks and in the evening, refuse to think about goals, projects, or tasks that are not part of the present moment. If a stressful thought comes to mind, choose to move on to a thought that is related to what you are presently seeing, hearing, smelling, or feeling.

If you have to stop at a red light while driving to work, don't get frustrated, but consider it a welcome opportunity to be thankful for your car, your job, your boss, and so on. The majority of people in third world countries would love to have your car, your job, and your boss. Quit complaining about what you don't have, and start practicing gratitude for what you do have. You can practice gratitude by enjoying the music, the sights around you, the fact that you have air conditioning or heating for your car or house, and the fact that you have a car and are well enough to drive.

As you practice mindfulness, your muscles will relax, your body unwinds, and your stress is relieved. I encourage my patients to take a drive in the country, take a walk, play with children or grandchildren, smell the flowers, or go to the zoo and look at the animals. This teaches them to get absorbed in the present moment so their minds can de-stress naturally.

My favorite way to practice mindfulness is taking my grandson Braden to the park. He is so excited and runs to the slide and slides down and then climbs back up the slide again. He then loves to stop and pick up wood chips on the ground and then stick them in any tiny little hole he finds, which is usually in the playground equipment. One day he sat for an hour near the top of the slide simply breaking off little twigs and sticking them through the small holes in the flooring of the playground equipment. He also loves to run and have me chase him, saying, "Papa, get me!" He gets so tickled that he falls to the ground. He then looks up in the sky and loves to see airplanes. But his favorite sight is seeing the moon every night. In watching Braden, I enjoy practicing mindfulness.

To have complete mental and physical health, mindfulness must become a way of life, a continual pattern for practicing relaxation during your day. Make mindfulness a habit by practicing it daily.

THANKFULNESS AND GRATITUDE

Nothing exemplifies mindfulness better than thankfulness and gratitude. It's interesting that the Bible says in Psalm 100:4 that you "enter his [God's] gates with thanksgiving," because an "attitude of gratitude" helps you take the focus off your situation and shift it to the One who can work everything out for you. Hebrews 13 tells us to give the sacrifice of praise continually, not just when we feel like it, "the fruit of our lips, giving thanks to His name" (Heb. 13:15, NKJV). Paul said, "In every thing give thanks [even in the midst of trials and tribulations]: for this is the will of God in Christ Jesus concerning you" (1 Thess. 5:18, KJV).

I often have my patients start a gratitude journal and put pictures of loved ones in it. You should do the same. Also put pictures of fun vacations, birthdays, anniversaries that were special, and plenty of fun memories. Then savor these memories as you close your eyes and replay them in your mind. You'll find yourself laughing as you relive and savor these special occasions. I recommend that you start each day by identifying at least twenty or thirty specific things, great and small, for which you are grateful. Do this with your family at the breakfast table; you can do it alone in the shower. Make it part of your running mental dialogue wherever you go. Practicing gratitude will "unstick" your stuck stress response, and it will induce a relaxation response in your body.

Thankfulness and mindfulness will go a long way toward erasing the stress in your life. You will enjoy each day of your life, and your tension and stress will be greatly reduced as you begin to live in the present moment instead of the past or future and as you give praise and thanksgiving to God every moment of the day. I also recommend ten belly laughs a day to all my patients since it relaxes the entire body and stress typically melts away.

CHANGE YOUR PERSPECTIVE THROUGH "REFRAMING"

Mindfulness is learning to live in the present moment. Reframing is learning to see the past, present, and future in a positive light. Reframing calls upon a person to shift his focus away from his present point of view in order to "see" another person or a situation from a new perspective.

Here's a simple example of the concept of reframing. We had a beautiful painting in our living room, but it was never noticed because the picture frame didn't do the painting justice. My wife finally decided to reframe it with a beautiful new frame. The result was amazing. It was as if the painting almost came alive, and practically everyone noticed it immediately upon entering the room. People who had been in my house dozens of times and never noticed it were now awestruck by its beauty. They would ask where we had purchased the remarkable new painting. I replied that we had the painting hanging there all along, but no one had ever noticed it until we changed the frame.

Yes, it's true that you cannot control everything that happens to you, but you can control your perceptions and interpretations of what happens. Any psychologist will tell you that your perceptions and reactions are more important to your mental and physical health than the event itself.

Every thought you have ripples throughout your entire being—your physical body and emotions. Stressful thoughts do damage to your body and mind, like a grenade going off. Proverbs 4:23 says, "Guard your heart above all else, for it determines the course of your life." According to Strong's concordance, *heart* in this verse is from the Hebrew word that means "the inner person, self; the seat of thoughts and emotion; conscience, mind, understanding." Romans 8:5–6 tells us, "Those who are dominated by the sinful nature think about sinful things, but those who are controlled by the Holy Spirit think about things that please the Spirit. So letting your sinful nature control your mind leads to death. But letting the Spirit control your mind leads to life and peace." The apostle Paul wrote in Philippians 2:5, "Let this mind be in you, which was also in Christ Jesus" (KJV).

If we allow the sinful nature to control our mind, it leads to death, but if we allow the Holy Spirit to control our mind, it leads to life and peace. We can also allow the mind of Jesus to be in us. But we must learn to think, act, and react the way Jesus did by walking in love and being full of the Holy Spirit and reframing every thought in line with the Word of God, according to 2 Corinthians 10:4–5. That means we must learn to reframe every event in our lives that we perceived as tragic, painful, traumatic, or in any way negative.

I knew one woman who had witnessed her father kill her mother with a gun. This woman spent many years trapped in anxiety and panic attacks, dwelling on the fact that her mother was killed in front of her. My wife finally told her, "Look at what God protected you from instead of what the enemy was successful at doing. You weren't killed that day. You were spared." That woman began to reframe her past and see it in a better light and, as a result, eventually overcame both her anxiety and the panic attacks.

Unfortunately, many people choose to relive the painful past experience. When their expectations are not met, even on small matters, they consider it a crisis of epic proportions. Because of the way they have been "programmed" to think either by their upbringing or by choice, they never break free and never begin to reframe events by God's standard of truth. But to cope with stress, we must recognize and "cast down" any perception that is contrary to the truth. His stress-management program is much better than what has been programmed into us since childhood.

Reframing is a concept pioneered by psychologist Albert Ellis, whose rational emotive therapy sought to help people replace irrational beliefs and perceptions with rational, realistic statements. When negative thoughts pop up spontaneously, Ellis said, you should challenge and assess them. Don't just accept them automatically.[2]

This is exactly what the apostle Paul meant by "casting down imaginations" and being "transformed by the renewing of your mind."

> *Casting down imaginations*, and every high thing that exalteth itself against the knowledge of God, and bringing into captivity every thought to the obedience of Christ.
> —2 Corinthians 10:5, kjv, emphasis added

> Do not be conformed to this world, but *be transformed by the renewing of your mind*, that you may prove what is that good and acceptable and perfect will of God.
> —Romans 12:2, nkjv, emphasis added

James, the brother of Jesus, taught us the meaning of reframing when we face trials:

> My brethren, count it all joy when you fall into various trials, knowing that the testing of your faith produces patience.
> —James 1:2–3, nkjv

James was giving us God's perspective. Scriptural reframing is one of the most powerful ways to relieve stress. It is simply replacing our fears, worries, failures, grief, sorrows, and shame with God's promises.

One woman I treated had been carjacked while at a phone booth at a service station. Two thugs almost raped her, but they didn't. They stole her brand-new car, which had her purse, driver's license, and home address. This woman had panic attacks because she knew the men had her identification that told them where she lived. She lived in fear that they would come back and rape her.

But the fact was they did not rape her, and they never came back for her. All she lost was her car and her purse, and the car was insured. She lost no money other than what was in her purse, but she lost her peace. I told her to reframe the event in her mind. Instead of reliving the traumatic experience, I encouraged her to start being grateful that she was protected from any harm. I said, "Let this be a lesson that angels encamp around you and stand guard to protect you."

She responded, "I've never seen it that way." As she reframed the event, the fear and anxiety resolved.

In reframing, see your trials as your teacher. I have found that practically all traumatic events can be reframed so that a lesson is learned and gratitude expressed.

The story of one Holocaust survivor, Dr. Viktor Frankl, a Jewish psychiatrist, is a powerful example of reframing. One day he was naked and alone in a small room, and it suddenly dawned on him that the "last of human freedom"—his inner identity—was the very freedom that his Nazi captors could not take away. This freedom was his inner identity and the power to choose how he would react. Frankl said humor was an essential part of his survival. Frankl also encouraged his fellow prisoners to tell at least one funny story every day about something that they intended to do after they were freed. Frankl was reframing his thoughts as well as helping his fellow prisoners reframe theirs. He understood the healing power of laughter and eventually went on to develop a school of psychotherapy called *logo thinking*, which incorporates humor as a major part of therapy.

I frame my day each morning, and I encourage you to do the same. Live each day as if it were your last. From eternity's perspective, even "big" problems seem small. James wrote, "You do not know what will happen tomorrow. For what is your life? It is even a vapor that appears for a little time and then vanishes away" (James 4:14, NKJV).

By staying mindful of the present, thankful to God, and by reframing everything that happens to you according to the truth of God's Word, you will be able to cope with the major sources of stress in your life.

PRACTICE TIME MANAGEMENT

Learning new ways of managing your time can dramatically reduce your stress as well. If you are forty years old, statistically you have used up more than half of your life on this earth. Have you ever stopped to reflect on how wise you've been in the management of that time? Learning to manage your time is critically important for conquering stress. Let's take a look at a few extremely important time management strategies.

Avoid time suckers

Do you know what a "sucker" is? Farmers know that trees must be pruned to cut off the suckers. These are large branches that grow out of control and tend to sap the tree of all of its energy and nourishment. When the farmer prunes his apple trees or pear trees, he cuts off those branches so the entire tree can be nourished in a balanced, healthy way.

This phenomenon also occurs in our lives with our time. We

all experience time suckers. These are activities, relationships, business ventures, and anything else that rob our lives of enormous amounts of time and energy to the point at which the overall health of our lives is depleted. Suckers drain us and pull us off of the path of health and godliness.

A sucker can be as simple as the onslaught of telemarketing calls you receive each evening at dinnertime that steals away your peaceful family moments. Or a sucker can be as major as a close relationship with a relative who is controlling and overbearing and who is stealing your family's harmony in order to meet his or her own needs through you.

One of the most important things you can do is to identify the time suckers in your life and take steps to eliminate or reduce their negative effect by making a commitment to stop giving in to their demands and manipulations and simply learning to say no. If you don't give in to their demands, they are no longer controlling you.

Get organized

Time is ultimately your most precious possession. How you spend your time determines, in many ways, how you will spend eternity. Many people stay stressed because they fail to organize their time. This is so simple to do, but some people don't know where to begin. I recommend these steps:

1. Purchase a calendar organizer, PDA, or access the calendar feature on your smart phone if you have one. Put key dates—such as birthdays and anniversaries, as well as appointments and the dates of major events—onto the calendar.

2. Organize your desk at work or home—the place where you do your paperwork, pay bills, and so forth. The average office worker spends about thirty-six hours a week at his desk and another three hours a week sorting piles trying to locate which project to work on next![3]

3. Throw away junk mail (and e-mail) daily.

4. Buy a filing cabinet or organizing system for storing important papers, articles, warranties, tax documents, deeds, wills, and other valuable items that may currently be stuck in various drawers throughout the house.

5. Organize your kitchen. Countless hours are spent searching for items in the kitchen as one prepares meals. Stay organized, and meal preparation will be easier and faster.

6. Prevent nuisance phone calls by telemarketers. Get caller ID, block these calls, or simply turn off your phone's ringer during certain hours to avoid taking calls that are a total waste of your time. I signed up to be on a "no call list" for marketers at www .donotcall.gov.

7. Declare one day a week, or perhaps one weekend a month, as media "fast" time. That means no Internet, no social media, no computer games, no video games, no iPods, no texting on cell phones, no DVDs, and no television. Use this time to connect with your family or friends. As a general rule, choose to cut back on your television-

watching time. In the average American home, the
television set is turned on for seven hours a day,
and the average viewer watches between twenty and
thirty-six hours of television a week.[4] Most of that
viewing is a total waste of time! If you think you
are watching television just for "escapism" or "fun,"
ask yourself what you are trying to escape from and
why you are looking for "fun" in the media rather
than being with people and creating your own
"fun."

8. Make the most of your "waiting" times. Everybody,
   even physicians, find themselves in waiting rooms
   from time to time. It may be a doctor's office or
   dentist office, an appointment at the DMV, bank,
   or airport. Always have a book, magazine, or music
   available to fill this time with something positive
   and productive. "Shouldn't I just chill out and
   relax?" you may ask. These environments are not
   places of relaxation—you may as well make good
   use of your time and do something productive!
   Taking a five- or ten-minute mini vacation in your
   mind is a good use of a "waiting" time, but most
   people find themselves waiting for longer periods.
   Have something positive to do.

9. Make a conscious decision to limit the amount of
   time you spend with negative, pessimistic people.
   They not only will sabotage your goals, but they
   will also drain energy from you. I call these people
   "energy vampires" or "energy leeches" because

no matter what you do, they seem to make you "tired" by their endless whining, complaining, and bickering. Avoid this frustration by avoiding or limiting your time spent with such people.

10. Refuse to be distracted if you are focused on a work project. Forward your phone calls to voice mail or have somebody answer your calls. Close your door. Don't allow for interruptions. You can generally get more done in an hour of totally focused time without interruptions than in three hours of time that has only a few interruptions.

    Individuals with type A personalities are prone to multitasking (doing more than one thing at a time). Focusing on just one thing at a time will take discipline. It requires doing fewer things. Stick with one task until it is finished, and then move on to the next.

11. Make a to-do list each evening before you go to bed. This way you don't need to continue to mull things over in your mind all night. You know the list is made and waiting for you in the morning. Once the list is made, refuse to think about it until morning. As part of your to-do list, set a specific time to exercise, have your daily devotional and prayer time, and eat your meals. Make sure you have a little "margin" for relaxation and for emergencies or unavoidable interruption. Remain flexible, and do not let interruptions unnerve you.

12. Make dining an enjoyable experience by tasting, smelling, and savoring every bite of food instead of wolfing it down. (This is the main reason why the French people have significantly fewer problems with obesity than Americans, even though they eat small portions of rich desserts and pastries.) I recommend that you give yourself at least thirty minutes to connect with family members. Do not scold or reprimand children at mealtime. Also, avoid arguments and stressful topics at mealtime.

Avoid eating on the run or as you drive your car. You need to be able to relax, chew every bite thirty times, and give your body's digestive system an opportunity to do its work. A great deal of stress can be eliminated if a person will simply use mealtimes as opportunities to relax, daydream a little, rest, and laugh.

I know some people who spend as much as two hours a day commuting to and from work. I recommend that these people use the CD player or auxiliary player in their vehicle to listen to audio books, take an audio college course, learn a new language, or expand their awareness of classical music. Choose to be a good steward of your time, and as a part of your stewardship, build in a healthy margin that is totally unscheduled. This time is likely to fuel your creativity and energy and defuse your stress level simultaneously.

Plan your work, and work your plan

Highly successful people will tell you that one of the most important keys to success is planning. The Bible says, "Where there is no vision, the people perish" (Prov. 29:18, KJV).

Have you prayerfully set goals for your life? Have you prayerfully created a plan for your business or ministry? Do you have a vision for exercise, diet, and health? Have you prayerfully developed a plan for reaching the objectives you feel are important? Careful, wise, and prayerful planning plays a vital role in reducing stress and helping you reach your objectives.

What is your purpose? Proverbs 19:21 says, "You can make many plans, but the LORD's purpose will prevail." Pray to know God's purpose for you. Start by following your passion!

Learn to delegate

I run a hectic medical practice, so occasionally I have a massage therapist come to our busy office to give a few of the staff a massage, which is also a great stress reliever. Often the massage therapist remarks how relaxed and unstressed my muscles are compared to others on staff whose muscles are knotted from stress. I believe this is because I've learned to delegate effectively, which allows me to accomplish a great deal without becoming overly stressed.

Learn to delegate; you don't have to do it all. If you don't have a good reason for doing a certain job or duty, then delegate it so that you will have time to do the things you enjoy and are most skilled at.

Build "margin" into your life

In his book *The Overload Syndrome*, Dr. Richard Swenson contends that margin is the difference between vitality and exhaustion. It is where we gain breathing room and store up reserve energy.[5] If you are always in a hurry or always tired, it's usually because you haven't built enough margin into your schedule.

When you live without enough margin in your time, finances, and so on, you become instantly stressed. You may be overstressed simply because you are too busy. It may be overcommitment, too many activities, compounded by a growing to-do list added to an already hectic schedule.

Some people are on a "do-more-so-I-can-have-more" treadmill. The more some people have, the more they want, and so the harder they work. Recognize that eventually those things will own you instead of you owning them because they will consume your time and energy. It will rob you of peace and joy. People begin to irritate you, and you may become critical or complain too much, which causes even more stress. Developing margin breaks you out of this trap.

I have read through the Bible a number of times, and I have noticed that Jesus was never in a hurry. He knew how to build margin into His life. We need to slow down and get into God's rhythm.

Margin will not magically appear in your schedule or finances. You must plan it and put it there. Some people should cut back on their commitments by learning to say no or by being less ambitious. Others have plenty of time in their schedules, but they manage it poorly and are chronically late anyway. I have seen license plate frames that read, "Always late, but worth the wait." That is a selfish attitude. You stress other people out by being late, and you steal the margin they have built into their schedules. Learn to be punctual. Make a to-do list each evening before you go to bed, and build in time between your appointments. It will decrease your stress and the stress of people who might have to wait on you.

Other people desperately need to build margin into their finances. A third of Americans say money is a very significant source of stress for them.[6] Financial advice is beyond the scope of this book, but the most basic is often the best: spend less than you earn, pay off credit cards each month, build an emergency fund equal to four to six months of pay, have health insurance, and get out of debt. These things protect you when unexpected expenditures hit.

I find a large percentage of people are stressed because they are caught up in materialism and the resulting debt. They compare what they have with their neighbors, relatives, employers, and friends, and they feel obligated to keep up with the Joneses. They buy a brand-new SUV, new clothes, new jewelry, a new home, new boat, and the newest electronic gadgets—and all on credit. The Word of God is clear on this: "Seek first the kingdom of God and His righteousness, and all these things shall be added to you" (Matt. 6:33, NKJV). I have also realized that the happiest and most joyful people I encounter as patients are not the richest or the ones who have the most things. They are the ones who invest their time and energy in people and not things. Learn to live within your financial means. Budget yourself and make a plan to get out of debt. Two sources I personally recommend are Dave Ramsey and Crown Financial Ministries. They are a good start to provide information on getting your finances in order. See Appendix B for more information.

When you have margin in your life, you will sometimes find yourself at the doctor's office or other appointments five minutes early instead of late. Make the most of your time by bringing along work, something to read, or something to listen to. When you intentionally build margin into your life, your stress level will go down dramatically.

Do it now!

Did you know that those who procrastinate often have a fear of rejection or failure, which causes them to put off accomplishing certain tasks? Determine that with God's help you will confront your fears, roll up your sleeves, and get busy.

Create a plan for accomplishing your tasks, and then slowly start chipping away at them one piece at a time. Once you have completed a particular job, reward yourself for a job well done.

All work and no play

Be sure your life has a healthy balance of work and play, difficult jobs and easy ones, tasks you enjoy and those you consider drudgery. All work and no play is unhealthy and will cause you to feel stressed out. If you work very hard, make sure you take vacations and short getaways. Balance is a key factor in health and happiness.

Clean off your plate

One reason you may be feeling overly stressed is because you have too much on your plate. You may have more debts, commitments, responsibilities, and demands than you are able to handle. If you are overextended, clear your plate.

Pay off your debts. Most of us can't do that all at once, but setting a plan in place to do so will eliminate a mountain of stress.

Stop volunteering for duties that you don't have time for.

You have a right to save some time for you. Don't get involved in more volunteer, school, church, or work activities or projects than you can easily and effectively handle. If you are feeling stressed out, back off a little until your life feels more in control.

Learning to say no is one of the most important things you can do to manage stress in your life. There's always someone who wants to borrow your car, your clothes, your money, your lawn mower, or who wants to fill up your days with their own cares and responsibilities. When you are unable to say no to a person's request, that person's problem has now become your problem, and his or her burden is now your burden.

Instead of churning in emotional circles of frustration and anger, simply say, "No, I can't. Send my greetings to everyone at home." No apologizing, no long explanations—just simply, politely say no and move on to another topic.

RECOGNIZE YOUR NEED FOR SLEEP

First and foremost we need to recognize that God designed our bodies to need sleep. We need this "down time" every night to restore, remove, and replace worn-out and dead cells in the body. We also need adequate sleep to give the brain an opportunity to "sort out" the information of the day in ways that are intricately designed by our Creator and are far too complex to begin to explain here. In extremely simplified terms, we need a sufficient break from sensory input in order to categorize and store information for use as "memories" that guide future behavior.

As part of recognizing that we need sleep, we must come to value sleep. A majority of Americans, however, don't seem to value sleep enough to get the sleep they need. Americans average a little less than seven hours of sleep a night, but sleep experts generally recommend seven to eight hours of sleep a night.[7] A National Sleep Foundation survey revealed that the majority of Americans—75 percent—had at least one symptom of a sleep problem, and 54 percent experienced at least one symptom of insomnia.[8] As a result, many Americans report "daytime drowsiness."

I recommend that a person try to find the root cause of the insomnia—such as excessive stress, depression, anxiety, or chronic pain—rather than resort to medication. For information on natural treatments for insomnia, please refer to my book *The New Bible Cure for Sleep Disorders.*

CONCLUSION

Don't let a mountain of stress avalanche down upon your life and health. There's so much you can do to conquer that mountain and rise to the top. God never intended for stress to rob your life of happiness and peace.

Why not determine right now to begin implementing these mental strategies for conquering stress. Living stressed out is not God's best for you. His wonderful Word says:

> Don't worry about anything; instead, pray about everything. Tell God what you need, and thank him for all he has done. Then you will experience God's peace, which exceeds anything we can understand. His peace will guard your hearts and minds as you live in Christ Jesus.
>
> —PHILIPPIANS 4:6–7

With God's help and some wise strategies, you can develop entirely new, stress-free ways of living your life.

A **BIBLE CURE** *Prayer for You*

Dear Lord, I give You all of my stress-producing ways of thinking and living. Renew my mind by helping me to develop and learn new lifestyle strategies so that I may enjoy greater productivity, happiness, and peace. In Jesus's name, amen.

A **BIBLE CURE** *Prescription*

List all the things you must do.

_____

_____

_____

List all the things you want to do.

_____

_____

_____

List the things you currently do that you neither want to do or must do.

_____

_____

_____

Draw a giant X over the items in the third list. These are the things you need to eliminate from your life in order to deal with stress. Develop a plan to eliminate or reduce all of these items in six months. Write out that plan.

_____

_____

_____

Chapter 5

SPIRITUAL STRATEGIES FOR COPING WITH STRESS

YOU CAN BEGIN to manage stress by developing a new belief system that sees God as the One who is in control of your life. The Bible says, "Seek ye first the kingdom of God, and his righteousness; and all these things shall be added unto you" (Matt. 6:33, KJV). God will add to your life the peace, happiness, and control that you need when you give Him first place.

How do you do this? You must abide in the vine. In other words, you must learn to see Jesus Christ as the complete and total source of your life. When you do so, you will be walking in the Spirit. Galatians 5:16–17 (NKJV) says:

> I say then: Walk in the Spirit, and you shall not fulfill the lust of the flesh. For the flesh lusts against the Spirit, and the Spirit against the flesh; and these are contrary to one another, so that you do not do the things that you wish.

Your mind acts like a referee choosing how you will receive and perceive the events of your life. Will you feel overwhelmed by them, or confident and in control no matter what happens?

If you get your mind on the side of the Spirit by filling it with God's Word, you will make the right choices and will rise above every negative, harmful, and stress-producing emotion.

REMOVING THE ROOTS OF STRESS

The Word of God is very powerful. It has the power to reprogram the way you think, causing your thinking to line up with God's way of seeing things. When you renew your mind with God's Word according to Romans 12:1–2, you begin to pull out stressful ways of thinking by their very roots. You are removing the old software package or old way of thinking and putting in God's software package. The Bible says, "Bringing every thought into captivity to the obedience of Christ" (2 Cor. 10:5, NKJV).

When my patients come to me with physical and emotional symptoms that are rooted in stress, I prescribe scriptures to help them renew their minds and confessions to activate their faith, along with a nutritional program to strengthen their bodies. Here's how it works.

If your mind tells you, "You'll never amount to anything," you can reprogram your mind with God's Word by responding as follows:

> God tells me in Deuteronomy 28:13 that the Lord will make me the head and not the tail. If I pay attention to the commands of the Lord my God and follow them, I will always be at the top and never at the bottom. I boldly confess that I always succeed

and prosper, and God's blessing and favor rest upon me.

At the end of this chapter I have prepared a Bible Cure prescription for you with God's Word that is specifically directed at your own personal roots of stress, your own stinking thinking. Whenever you hear your own mind speak negative, stress-producing thoughts, you can reprogram it with these verses I have provided to yank your stress up by the roots. It is also important to confess this out of your mouth on a regular basis.

In addition, here are some more keys to renewing your mind with God's Word.

Practice Forgiveness

Many people harbor hidden anger, bitterness, unforgiveness, resentment, fear, hatred, abandonment, shame, and rejection and aren't even aware of it. What about you? Do memories of old wounds and hurts surface in your thoughts when you encounter certain people? Have you been hurt in the past and simply buried the hurt? Feelings buried alive never die.

Holding on to unforgiveness doesn't punish the individual who wronged you. It only destroys you through the roots of stress. I once heard a person say that bitterness was like drinking poison and wishing someone else would die. Mark 11:25 says, "But when you are praying, first forgive anyone you are holding a grudge against, so that your Father in heaven will forgive your sins, too." But you say, "That's not fair; you don't know how badly they hurt me, slandered me, betrayed me, rejected me." It's not an issue of being fair but of being obedient to God's Word. God knows how damaging unforgiveness is to us mentally, emotionally, physically, and spiritually. Ephesians 4:31–32 says, "Get rid of all bitterness, rage, anger, harsh words, and slander, as well as all types of evil behavior. Instead, be kind to each other, tenderhearted, forgiving one another, just as God through Christ has forgiven you."

I am leaving you with a gift—peace of mind and heart.

—JOHN 14:27

DIVINE FORGETFULNESS

Not only do you need to forgive those who have hurt and offended you, but you also need to forget it. "Forgetting those things which are behind and reaching forward to those things which are ahead, I press toward the goal for the prize of the upward call of God in Christ Jesus" (Phil. 3:13–14, NKJV).

LEARN TO LOVE

First Corinthians 13:8 says, "Love never fails" (NKJV). Are you in a political battle at work? Do you have strife in your family? Have you been hurt by your spouse? Love truly never fails—and it will not fail you! Can you imagine, there is only one thing the Bible tells us will never fail us, and that is practicing the love walk. We need to practice all the characteristics of love in 1 Corinthians 13:4–7. I recommend reading this passage aloud and inserting yourself in place of love in these verses.

Love is patient and kind. [I am patient and kind.]
Love is not jealous or boastful or proud or rude. [I
am not jealous or boastful or proud or rude.] It does
not demand its own way. [I do not demand my own
way.] It is not irritable, and it keeps no record of
being wronged. [I am not irritable, and I keep no
record of being wronged.] It does not rejoice about
injustice but rejoices whenever the truth wins out. [I
do not rejoice about injustice but rejoice whenever
the truth wins out.] Love never gives up, never
loses faith, is always hopeful, and endures through
every circumstance. [I never give up, never lose
faith, am always hopeful, and endure through every
circumstance.]

Notice that love keeps no record of wrongs. In other words,
forgiveness is part of love. Throw away the record-keeping book
and forgive everyone who has wronged you. As Christians
there is only one commandment we have, and it is the love
commandment. (See John 13:34.)

Fear rules the lives of many people, but the Bible says, "Perfect
love expels all fear" (1 John 4:18). You can live free from fear as
you increasingly understand the power of God's love for you.
Mahatma Gandhi said that the whole world would accept the
Christ of Christians if the Christians would only act like Christ.

Build and maintain the ties of relationships. Relationships
with those who love you are gifts from God. Never take them
for granted!

LEARN TO LAUGH

The Bible says, "A cheerful heart is good medicine" (Prov. 17:22). If you are stressed out, why not take a prescription for laughter? When you're down or stressed, pick up a wholesome, funny video and watch it. A good, strong twenty-second belly laugh is equivalent to three minutes on a rowing machine, according to one study.[1] Laughter releases tension, anxiety, anger, fear, shame, and guilt, and it can transform your attitude and outlook.

When people come into my office to be treated or placed on a nutritional program, I often ask them, "How often do you laugh?" You should see the looks they give me. A common response in cancer patients is, "I never laugh." I can tell they're thinking, "I have cancer, Dr. Colbert. What is there to laugh about?"

One of the most unusual prescriptions I give to many of my patients is to have at least ten belly laughs a day, with each belly laugh lasting at least twenty seconds. True laughing offers one of the most powerful and natural healing methods without any side effects. Laughter lowers the stress hormones cortisol and epinephrine. It increases feel-good hormones. It keeps you squarely in the present moment practicing mindfulness. It helps you to reframe and feel thankful and helps you to see negative events in a more positive light. There's not a single bad thing laughter will do for your body and mind.

BENEFITS OF HAPPINESS

According to Rich Bayer, PhD, CEO of Upper Bay Counseling and Support Services, Inc., happy people have more social contact and better social relations than their unhappy counterparts.

Studies of positive people show that they rate high on having good relationships with themselves and with others. Their love for life is better as well. Happy people tend to be kinder to others and to express empathy more easily.

Of course, happy people are not "luckier" than other people. They experience their share of tragedy and hardship, but studies show that they do a better job of reframing.[2] They remember the good events in their lives more readily, and when bad things happen, they believe things will eventually be all right. They have hope.

Happiness is one of the keys to a long, satisfying life. Studies also show that happy people have fewer health problems.[3] Research among older people indicates that folks with positive emotions outlive their sour counterparts. Happy people were shown to be half as likely to become disabled as sad people in the same age bracket. And happy people have a higher pain threshold than those who are sad.[4]

When you laugh, powerful chemicals called endorphins, which act much the same way as morphine, are released in the brain. Endorphins trigger a feeling of well-being throughout your entire body and relieve pain.

In the Department of Behavioral Medicine of the UCLA Medical School, a man named Norman Cousins conducted extensive research into the physical benefits of happiness. He established the Humor Research Task Force, which coordinated worldwide clinical research on humor. His research proved conclusively that laughter, happiness, and joy are perfect antidotes for stress.[5]

A good hearty laugh can:

- Decrease stress hormones, which helps you relax
- Improve quality of sleep
- Relieve pain
- Lower blood pressure
- Boost the immune system
- Enhance brain function
- Increase longevity
- Protect the heart and prevent heart attack
- Connect you to others
- Prevent divorce
- Elevate mood and help relieve anxiety and depression
- Work similar to exercise

According to the Association for Applied and Therapeutic Humor, "Without humor one's thought processes are likely to become stuck and narrowly focused, leading to increased distress."[6]

Choosing a good attitude doesn't diminish the amount of suffering in your life or in the world, but it helps to lighten the load. Even when we suffer, we can choose to be joyful because God is with us.

Dr. Lee Berk and fellow researcher Dr. Stanley Tan of Loma Linda University in California studied the effects of laughter on the immune system and found a general decrease in stress hormones that constrict blood vessels and suppress immune activity in people exposed to humor. Levels of the stress hormone epinephrine were lower in the group both in anticipation of humor and after exposure to humor. Epinephrine levels remained down throughout the experiment.[7]

As I stated earlier, I recommend to all my patients ten belly laughs a day. I prescribe Carol Burnett DVDs, *Sanford and Son* DVDs, and other clean humor to my patients. Create a habit of happiness instead of a habit of worry. Your happiness is not at the mercy of other people or life circumstances and events. A merry heart is your greatest weapon against stress. For more information on this topic, please refer to my books *Deadly Emotions* and *Stress Less*.

A **BIBLE CURE** Prayer for You

Dear heavenly Father, I come before Your throne asking for Your power for a brand-new mind, completely transformed by Your mighty and wonderful Word. I submit my life to You, and I ask You to change the way I think and feel. Let my mind line up with the ways that You think. Let my heart rise up in new faith and love. Restore and heal my body from the ravages of stress. Strengthen and renew me completely so that I can walk in Your light and extend Your love to a stressed-out, weary world. In Jesus's name, amen.

A **BIBLE CURE** Prescription

Below you will find some negative thoughts and scriptures that directly uproot those stressful thoughts. Select the verses that are most appropriate to you, and write them down on index cards. Speak them aloud three times a day—at breakfast, lunch, and bedtime.

"I'm a failure and a loser." —Romans 8:37; Philippians 4:13

"I'm worthless and pitiful." —2 Corinthians 6:16; Galatians 4:7; Ephesians 2:10

"I'm no good." —2 Corinthians 5:17

"I'm stupid and dumb." —1 Corinthians 1:30; 2:16; James 1:5

"I'm unattractive." —1 Samuel 16:7; Romans 5:5; Ephesians 2:10

"I'm not teachable." —Psalm 32:8

"I'm a burden." —Deuteronomy 28:8

"I'm trapped." —John 8:32, 36

"I'm alone." —Matthew 28:20; Hebrews 13:5

"I'm guilty." —Psalm 103:12; Romans 8:1; 1 John 1:9

"I'm incapable." —Philippians 4:13

"I'm sinful." —John 3:14–18; 5:24

A Personal Note

FROM DON COLBERT

GOD DESIRES TO heal you of disease. His Word is full of promises that confirm His love for you and His desire to give you His abundant life. His desire includes more than physical health for you; He wants to make you whole in your mind and spirit as well through a personal relationship with His Son, Jesus Christ.

If you haven't met my best friend, Jesus, I would like to take this opportunity to introduce Him to you. It is very simple. If you are ready to let Him come into your life and become your best friend, all you need to do is sincerely pray this prayer:

> *Lord Jesus, I want to know You as my Savior and Lord. I believe You are the Son of God and that You died for my sins. I also believe You were raised from the dead and now sit at the right hand of the Father praying for me. I ask You to forgive me for my sins and change my heart so that I can be Your child and live with You eternally. Thank You for Your peace. Help me to walk with You so that I can begin to know You as my best friend and my Lord. Amen.*

If you have prayed this prayer, you have just made the most important decision of your life. I rejoice with you in your decision and your new relationship with Jesus. Please contact my publisher at pray4me@charismamedia.com so that we can send you some materials that will help you become established in your relationship with the Lord. We look forward to hearing from you.

Appendix A

CONFESSIONS FOR FAVOR AND FINANCIAL BLESSINGS

IRST LET ME explain the principle of faith; Hebrews 11:6 tell us that without faith it is impossible to please God. God said, "Let the weak say, 'I am strong'" (Joel 3:10, NKJV). He didn't say let the weak talk about their weakness. We're not supposed to talk about the way we are. We are supposed to talk about the way we want to be. Get in agreement with God. I can't talk of sickness and expect health. I can't speak defeat and expect victory. Nothing happens unless we speak. Release your faith with your words. When you speak faith, you get in agreement with God; but when you speak defeat, you get in agreement with the enemy. Don't talk *about* your problems; talk *to* your problems. When I say what God says about me, God has promised He will do it. Scripture says, "Let the redeemed of the Lord say so" (Ps. 107:2, NKJV). It doesn't say "think so" or "believe so." Something supernatural happens when I speak it out. I refuse to put my faith in my fears. Fear says, "Believe the negative." Faith says, "Believe the positive." Both fear and faith ask us to believe something we cannot see.

Read the following confessions aloud one to two times daily.

1. Father, You said the path of the righteous gets brighter and brighter; You said no good thing will You withhold because I walk uprightly; You said because I delight myself in You, You would give me the desires of my heart.

2. God is a God of increase, not decrease. He never wants us to go backward, only forward.

3. Psalm 102:13 says there is a set time for favor. I have entered my season of favor.

4. God has already lined up the right people, the right opportunities, and the right breaks that I need.

5. I declare that every gift, every talent, every dream, and every desire will come to pass, and I will overcome every obstacle and will fulfill my God-given destiny.

6. Father, I'm asking You to bless me so much that I can be a blessing to others.

7. God is my source, and I am connected to the vine. I will not just survive; I will thrive.

8. Father, You said Your favor will last for a lifetime, and You said goodness and mercy will follow me all the days of my life.

9. I have God's favor, and He is directing my steps. Whatever I touch will prosper and succeed.

10. Father, thank You that I have Your favor on my life. Thank You for directing my steps and causing me to be at the right place at the right time.

11. God says I will lend and not borrow. I boldly declare I am blessed. God is supplying all of my needs, and I have more than enough.

12. Father, thank You that Your favor surrounds me like a shield. Your favor is opening up doors that no man can shut. Your favor brings supernatural opportunities and divine connections, and it causes me to be at the right place at the right time.

13. I declare the rest of my life will be better than the first part of my life.

14. I declare I'm blessed, I'm prosperous, and God's favor surrounds me.

15. I announce to my debt, "It's finished." I announce to my house payment, "It is finished." My house is paid off, and my cars are paid off. I am debt free, and I owe no man.

16. God says I am coming out of debt and I'm coming into overflow. I see supernatural increase, supernatural promotion, and explosive blessings.

17. This is my year for supernatural opportunities and to see the fulfillment of my dreams.

18. I declare it is my season for abundance in health, abundance of prosperity, abundance in finance, abundance of good breaks, an abundance of favor, and abundance of creative ideas.

19. God has already lined up the right people, the right opportunities, and the right breaks that I need.

20. I have an attitude of faith, expectancy, praise, and thanksgiving.

21. New seasons have opened up in my life, and my set time of favor is here.

22. I have God's DNA in me, and I will fulfill my God-given destiny.

23. I declare that every gift, every talent, every dream, and every desire that God has put in me will come to pass.

24. I will overcome every obstacle and fulfill my purpose and my destiny.

25. God is able to do in me exceedingly and abundantly above all I can ask or think.

26. God, I'm asking for Your favor today, for supernatural opportunities, and that You would bring every dream and desire to fulfillment.

27. Like Jabez, I'm asking for Your favor, for Your increase, and for Your blessings in my life.

28. I am totally out of debt and owe no man.

29. Tremendous financial blessings are coming my way.

30. I am blessed, prosperous, creative, talented, and highly favored.

31. My greatest accomplishments are out in front of me.

32. I am filled with the knowledge of His will in all wisdom and spiritual understanding.

33. Now I hold fast to my confession of faith, and I remain in an attitude of gratitude thanking God for favor and financial blessings on my life.

RESOURCES FOR STRESS

Please mention Dr. Colbert as the referring physician for the companies below.

Divine Health Nutritional Products

1908 Boothe Circle
Longwood, FL 32750
Phone: (407) 331-7007
Website: www.drcolbert.com
E-mail: info@drcolbert.com

B-Complex Vitamins
B Complex Plus

Vitamin C
Divine Health Vitamin C

Glutathione Boosters
Max One (one capsule two times daily)
Max GXL (three capsules two times daily)
Max ATP

Magnesium
Divine Health Chelated Magnesium

Adaptogens
Divine Health Stress Manager
Stress Relief Drops
Relora (magnolia bark)

Amino Acids
Divine Health Serotonin Max
Divine Health L-Theanine

Adrenal Rebuilder
Adrenal Support
DSF (De-stress formula)

Adrenal Hormones
Divine Health Pregnenolone
Divine Health DHEA

Supplements from Don Colbert, MD
1908 Boothe Circle
Longwood, FL 32750
Phone: (407) 331-7007

Pregnenolone PleoLyposome Cream

DHEA PleoLyposome Cream

Myers IV for Adrenal
To find a doctor to administer this IV treatment, refer to www.worldhealth.net; some of the physicians listed there are trained in this protocol.

Metagenics
Phone: (800) 692-9400
Website: www.drcolbert.meta-ehealth.com
Refer to Dr. Don Colbert, #@7741, when ordering.

Cordyceps
Adreset

Crown Financial Ministries

P. O. Box 100
Gainesville, GA 30503-0100
Phone: (800) 722-1976
Website: www.crown.org

Dave Ramsey

The Lampo Group
1749 Mallory Lane
Brentwood, TN 37027
Phone: (888) 227-3223
Website: www.daveramsey.com

NOTES

INTRODUCTION
A BRAND-NEW BIBLE CURE FOR A BRAND-NEW YOU!

1. American Psychological Association, "Mind/Body Health: Did You Know?", http://www.apa.org/helpcenter/mind-body.aspx (accessed January 20, 2011).

2. American Institute of Stress, "America's No. 1 Health Problem," http://www.stress.org/americas.htm (accessed January 20, 2011).

3. Anne Fisher, "Stressed Out: Are We Having Fun Yet?", *Fortune*, October 1996, 224, referenced in Shane Blahunka, "Stress Management and You," University of St. Francis, http://www.stfrancis.edu/content/ba/ghkickul/stuwebs/btopics/works/stress.htm (accessed January 20, 2011).

4. American Institute of Stress, "Job Stress," http://www.stress.org/job.htm (accessed January 20, 2011).

5. Ibid.

CHAPTER 1
UNDERSTANDING THE ROOTS OF STRESS

1. American Psychological Association "Stress in America," October 24, 2007, 6.

2. T. H. Holmes and R. H. Rahe, "The Social Readjustment Rating Scale," *Journal of Psychosomatic Research* 11, no. 2 (1967): 213–218. Used by permission.

CHAPTER 2
SUPPLEMENT STRATEGIES FOR COPING WITH STRESS

1. A. Fidanza, "Therapeutic Action of Pantothenic Acid," *International Journal for Vitamin and Nutrition Research* 24, suppl (1983): 53–67.

2. Alfred H. Merrill Jr. and J. Michael Henderson, "Diseases Associated With Defects in Vitamin B_6 Metabolism or Utilization," *Annual Review of Nutrition* 7 (July 1987): 135–156.

3. Ralph Carmel, "Subtle Cobalamin Deficiency," *Annals of Internal Medicine* 124, no. 3 (February 1, 1996): 338–340.

4. Tufts University, "Getting Enough B_{12}?", E-News, September 10, 2001, http://enews.tufts.edu/stories/1263/2001/09/10/GettingEnoughB12/ (accessed January 21, 2011).

5. S. P. Stabler, J. Lindenbaum, and R. H. Allen, "Vitamin B_{12} Deficiency in the Elderly: Current Dilemmas," *American Journal of Clinical Nutrition* 66 (October 1997): 741–749.

6. A. Odumosu, "Ascorbic Acid and Cortisol Metabolism in Hypovitaminosis C Guinea Pigs," *International Journal for Vitamin and Nutrition Research* 52, no. 2 (1982): 176–185.

7. S. P. Campbell, "Vitamin C Lowers Stress Hormone in Rats," *Science News* 156, no. 10 (September 4, 1999): 158.

8. Mark Hyman, "Glutathione: The Mother of All Antioxidants," HuffingtonPost.com, April 10, 2010, http://www.huffingtonpost.com/ dr-mark-hyman/glutathione-the-mother-of_b_530494.html (accessed January 26, 2011).

9. Michael Lam, "Magnesium and Aging," LamMD.com, http://www .drlam.com/articles/1999-No3-MagnesiumandAging.asp (accessed January 25, 2011).

10. Center for Magnesium Education and Research, "Magnesium in Refined vs. Whole Foods," http://www.centerformaged.org/index.php?page =Mag+in+Refined+vs+Whole+Food (accessed January 21, 2011).

11. R. R. Engel et al., "Double-Blind Crossover Study of PS versus Placebo in Patients With Early Dementia of the Alzheimer Type," *European Neuropsychopharmacology* 2 (1999): 149–155.

12. P. Monteleone et al., "Blunting by Chronic PS Administration of the Stress-Induced Activation of the Hypothalamo-Pituitary-Adrenal Axis in Healthy Men," *European Journal of Clinical Pharmacology* 42, no. 4 (1992): 385–388.

13. K. Kuribara, W. B. Stavinoha, and Y. Maruyama, "Honokiol, a Putative Anxiolityc Agent Extracted From Magnolia Bark, Has No Diazepam-Like Side Effects in Mice," *Journal of Pharmacy and Pharmacology* 51, no. 1 (1999): 97–103.

14. H. Juribara et al., "The Anxiolytic Effect of Two Oriental Herbal Drugs in Japan Attributed to Honokio From Magnolia Bark," *Journal of Pharmacy and Pharmacology* 52, no. 11 (2000): 1425–1429.

15. Y. C. Lo et al., "Magnolon and Honokiol Isolated From Magnolia Officinalis Protect Rat Heart Mitochondria Against Lipid Peroxidation," *Biochemical Pharmacology* 47, no. 3 (1994): 549–553.

16. W. Poeldinger, B. Calanchini, and W. Schwarz, "A Functional-Dimensional Approach to Depression: Serotonin Deficiency as a Target

Syndrome in a Comparison of 5-Hydroxytryptophan and Fluvoxamine," *Psychopathology* 24, no. 2 (1991): 53–81.

CHAPTER 3
EXERCISE STRATEGIES FOR COPING WITH STRESS

1. Trevor Powell, *Free Yourself From Harmful Stress* (New York: DJ Publishing, 1997), 128.

2. Ibid., 129.

CHAPTER 4
MENTAL STRATEGIES FOR COPING WITH STRESS

1. Harvard Health Publications, "Mindfulness in a Hectic World," May 2009, http://www.health.harvard.edu/newsletters/Harvard_Heart_Letter/2009/May/Mindfulness-in-a-hectic-world (accessed January 24, 2011).

2. Albert Ellis, "REBT," http://www.rebt.ws/REBT%20explained.htm (accessed January 24, 2011).

3. Richard A. Swenson, *The Overload Syndrome* (Colorado Springs, CO: NavPress, 1998), 142.

4. Ibid., 155.

5. Ibid., 15.

6. *Medical News Today*, "Money Is Number One Cause of Stress Say Americans," April 1, 2004, http://www.medicalnewstoday.com/articles/6934.php (accessed January 24, 2011).

7. Lawrence J. Epstein with Steven Mardon, *The Harvard Medical School Guide to a Good Night's Sleep* (New York: McGraw-Hill, 2007), 5.

8. D. J. Buysse, L. Finn, and T. Young, "Onset, Remission, Persistence, and Consistency of Insomnia Symptoms Over 10 Years: Longtitudinal Results From the Wisconsin Sleep Cohort Study (WSCS)," *Sleep* 27, no. A268, abstract 602.

CHAPTER 5
SPIRITUAL STRATEGIES FOR COPING WITH STRESS

1. W. F. Fry et al., *Make 'Em Laugh* (Palo Alto, CA: Science and Behavior Books, 1972).

2. Rich Bayer, "Benefits of Happiness," Upper Bay Counseling and Support Services, Inc., http://www.upperbay.org/articles/benefits%20 of%20happiness.pdf (accessed January 24, 2011).

3. Ibid.

4. Ibid.

5. Norman Cousins, *Head First: The Biology of Hope and the Healing Power of the Human Spirit* (New York: Penguin, 1990), referenced in P. Wooten, "An Antidote for Stress," *Holistic Nursing Practice* 10, no. 2 (1996): 49–56.

6. Steven M. Sultanoff, "What Is Humor?", Association for Applied and Therapeutic Humor, http://www.aath.org/articles/art_sultanoff01.html (accessed January 24, 2011).

7. HolisticOnline.com, "Therapeutic Benefits of Laughter," http://www .holisticonline.com/humor_therapy/humor_therapy_benefits.htm (accessed January 24, 2011).

Don Colbert, MD, was born in Tupelo, Mississippi. He attended Oral Roberts School of Medicine in Tulsa, Oklahoma, where he received a bachelor of science degree in biology in addition to his degree in medicine. Dr. Colbert completed his internship and residency with Florida Hospital in Orlando, Florida. He is board certified in family practice and anti-aging medicine and has received extensive training in nutritional medicine.

If you would like more
information about natural and
divine healing, or information about
Divine Health nutritional products,
you may contact Dr. Colbert at:

DON COLBERT, MD
1908 Boothe Circle
Longwood, FL 32750
Telephone: 407-331-7007 (for ordering products only)
Website: www.drcolbert.com.

Disclaimer: Dr. Colbert and the staff of Divine Health Wellness Center are prohibited from addressing a patient's medical condition by phone, facsimile, or e-mail. Please refer questions related to your medical condition to your own primary care physician.

Pick up these great Bible Cure books by Don Colbert, MD:

The Bible Cure for ADD and Hyperactivity
The Bible Cure for Allergies
The Bible Cure for Arthritis
The Bible Cure for Asthma
The Bible Cure for Autoimmune Diseases
The Bible Cure for Back Pain
The Bible Cure for Candida and Yeast Infections
The Bible Cure for Colds, Flu and Sinus Infections
The Bible Cure for Headaches
The Bible Cure for Heartburn and Indigestion
The Bible Cure for Hepatitis and Hepatitis C
The Bible Cure for High Blood Pressure
The Bible Cure for High Cholesterol
The Bible Cure for Irritable Bowel Syndrome
The Bible Cure for Memory Loss
The Bible Cure for Menopause
The Bible Cure for PMS and Mood Swings
The Bible Cure for Prostate Disorders
The Bible Cure for Skin Disorders
The Bible Cure for Thyroid Disorders
The Bible Cure for Weight Loss and Muscle Gain
The Bible Cure Recipes for Overcoming Candida
The New Bible Cure for Chronic Fatigue and Fibromyalgia
The New Bible Cure for Depression and Anxiety
The New Bible Cure for Diabetes
The New Bible Cure for Cancer
The New Bible Cure for Heart Disease
The New Bible Cure for Osteoporosis
The New Bible Cure for Sleep Disorders
The New Bible Cure for Stress